In *Don't Choose a Cosmetic Surgeon Without Me*, Dr. Barry Lycka shares his insights on what makes a great cosmetic surgeon and how to find one. His keen vision sees truths that I recognize from 20 years of being around, interacting with, and being a plastic surgeon. If you are a considering choosing a surgeon, follow Dr Lycka's advice and don't chose one without him.

Dr. Daryl K. Hoffman, MD
Adjunct Clinical Faculty,
Division of Plastics Reconstructive Surgery,
Stanford University

Dr. Lycka is a master physician whose expertise is sought by patients and physicians from all over the world. Many wish to do great things in medicine, Barry does them. As a teacher his mentoring has been invaluable. The information in this book should become the bedrock of advice for anyone interested in aesthetic medicine. It is coming from a star amongst stars. Treat it like he is sitting in the room with you.

Charles E. Crutchfield III, MD
Clinical Professor of Dermatology
University of Minnesota

Don't Choose a Cosmetic Surgeon Without Me has really hit the nail on the head. Dr. Lycka has an very astute insight into the cosmetic surgery world that is a 'must read' for anyone considering cosmetic surgery. No where else can you get the real inside story that Dr Lycka provides in helping the consumer understand the intricacies of cosmetic surgery and in selecting the right cosmetic surgeon for the right procedure. Thousands of patients have spent hundreds of thousands of dollars on cosmetic procedures only to be disappointed in the results or upset with the lack of compassion from their cosmetic surgeon when all was said and done. By reading this book the patient can develop the critical ability to find the right cosmetic surgeon to meet his/her needs. I strongly recommend every patient read Dr Lycka's outstanding book before having any cosmetic procedure.

Jeffrey Riopelle, MD
Laser Advantage of San Ramon Medical Group,
San Ramon, CA

The patient or consumer can be confused with the types of cosmetic procedures, anti-aging treatments and the topical cosmetic treatments that currently exist. This new book can help the consumer make wise choices in deciding on the type of physician and the types of treatments that are best for them. Trying to decide which resurfacing procedure, which filler and which tightening procedure can be difficult without this background knowledge. Whether or not to undergo a non-invasive procedure to prevent an invasive procedure requires knowledge. I strongly recommend *Don't Choose a Cosmetic Surgeon Without Me* to anyone who needs more knowledge about cosmetic treatments.

Ron Moy, MD
Past President, American Academy of Dermatology
Professor, David Geffen School of Medicine at UCLA

DON'T CHOOSE A COSMETIC SURGEON WITHOUT ME

Your Complete Guide to Finding the Perfect Cosmetic Doctor

DON'T CHOOSE A COSMETIC SURGEON WITHOUT ME

Your Complete Guide to Finding the Perfect Cosmetic Doctor

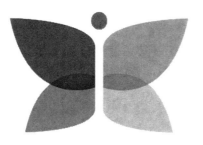

BARRY LYCKA M.D.

encompass
EDITIONS

Published by Encompass Editions, Kingston, Ontario, Canada. No part of this book may be reproduced, copied or used in any form or manner whatsoever without written permission, except for the purposes of brief quotations in reviews and critical articles.

For reader comments, orders, press and media inquiries:
www.encompasseditions.com

First edition 2013

ISBN: 978-0-9880428-9-6

Cataloguing in Publication Program (CIP) information available from
Library and Archives Canada at www.collectionscanada.gc.ca

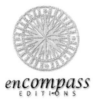

*en***compass**
EDITIONS

For the love of my life

The QR Codes

𝒯he internet has provided us with so many remarkable tools, I can't neglect it. Throught this book, you'll see here and there the perhaps familiar geometry of the QR code. If you have a smart phone or tablet device with a QR reader app, just scan the coded image and you'll be whisked off to on-line broadcasts, interviews and web sites that will deepen your knowledge of cosmetic surgery today.

Also by Dr. Barry Lycka

Shaping a New Image: The Practice of Cosmetic Surgery
More Shaping
Restoring YOUth: How to Recover and Keep Your Skin's Beauty
SkinWorks: How to Restore and Keep Your Natural Beauty

In Appreciation

I am always indebted to the many others from whom I draw inspiration and information for my books. It's truer than ever this time, when so many distinguished physicians have given me their time and shared their perspectives, and so many patients have volunteered their impressions and shared their experiences. I am truly grateful to you all.

FOREWORD

*S*ociety is incredibly unforgiving when it comes to aging in women, particularly when they are on television and in the public eye. Somehow women's knowledge and experience take a back seat when male decision-makers are choosing who is most "pleasing" to viewers to read the news, host our television shows or grace our magazine covers. Thankfully women over forty now have options in choosing treatments and services from dermatologists and plastic surgeons without the stigma of "having work done."

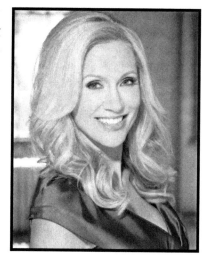

Wendi Russo
Television Personality and
Host with Shop NBC

Yet during this age of advancement in extending our looks beyond our mothers' or grandmothers' ability, we can find ourselves adrift in a sea of options with no resources other than friends willing to divulge their secrets, or gossip magazines revealing before-and-after photos of celebrities whose recent "work" has changed them significantly. What can we do to get our bearings?

Dr. Barry Lycka's newest book is comprehensive in educating us about the types of certifications now available and the lack of consistency in this field. He guides us towards an educated choice as to which doctor to use for which services. This can be, in my opinion, one of our most important decisions. An improperly executed cosmetic procedure—a less-than-natural lip, say, as the result of over-injection—can result in a woman not recognizing herself in the mirror. The effect can be devastating and sometimes irreversible.

I had my first baby at thirty-eight and at the age of forty-one, I entered my first beauty pageant because I thought it would motivate me to get back in shape. I was disappointed not to make the top five. It seemed I had to recognize that I could no longer compete in the realm of beauty with girls in their 20s and 30s. No one over forty had ever won our state's pageant.

I decided to focus on my fitness and nutrition, learn skills I hadn't realized I needed on stage and—this is important—visit a cosmetic dermatologiest, Dr. Charles Crutchfield III. The following year, I entered the pageant again and won. I was soon to realize the impact I, a titleholder, could make on children in my community. I re-competed a few years later and won Mrs. Minnesota United States, placing first runner up at the national pageant. With age comes experience and it is up to us to define our own limitations rather than allow society to place them upon us.

On a recent trip to Italy, my husband's family commented on how youthful I appeared. They guessed me to be in my thirties! I attribute this to genes, not smoking, eating right, exercising, not getting much sun—and Dr. Crutchfield. Like his friend and colleague Dr. Lycka, Dr. Crutchfield's natural choices—his "tweaking" as he calls it—has extended my youthful appearance and helped me feel more confident in the highly competitive field of television hosting. I'm not interested in erasing time and all wrinkles, but I do feel better seeing myself in the studio monitors and not noticing deep lines around my mouth or eyes.

Finding a doctor such as Dr. Crutchfield or Dr. Lycka is one of the wisest things we can do to maintain our looks. Their recommendations, years of experience and ability to listen to their patients' needs and concerns are important factors to consider when you're choosing a physician for any cosmetic procedure. "Don't choose a cosmetic surgeon without me!" Dr. Lycka says, and this little book gives you the tools you need to make the choices that will lead to a positive result. I encourage you to trust your instincts as you gain the knowledge you need. This will help you love the results you achieve.

Wishing you my best in your search!

Sincerely

Wendi Russo

INTRODUCTION

You've been thinking about having a cosmetic procedure done. You've seen programs about it on television. You've talked to friends who've had work done or at the very least they know someone else who has. You reasonably assume that it's a fairly straightforward business. It couldn't be more complicated than having a hernia repaired, could it? A lot less serious, in fact. You just need a referral to a good doctor and then make an appointment. No government or private insurance program is going to pay for it, so you also want a good price.

Maybe in some simpler world it is like that, but not in this one. When you decide on a cosmetic procedure you enter a labyrinth of decisions. It's not that there are no signs to point you this way or that: that would be some sort of natural labyrinth. This is a man-made labyrinth and there are signs everywhere. "Turn here!" "No! Go this way!" "Be careful! Don't go that way!" "Go *this* way, I said!"

When you have your hernia repaired, the surgeon your doctor refers you to is certified by the governing board of surgeons in your jurisdiction. Only certified practitioners are licensed to perform the surgery and no proper hospital would allow an unqualified surgeon to cut into your abdomen. But what if there was no clear standard for hernia repairs? What if there were no training standards? What if new techniques for repairing hernias were being constantly introduced? What if instead of a single certification board there were many—or none?

Welcome to the wonderful world of cosmetic medicine, where every practitioner—novice or veteran—is in some sense a pioneer pushing into new territory. And you are that territory.

The Canadian Society of Plastic Surgeons assures us that "Plastic Surgeons are the experts in cosmetic surgery." But the

American Board of Cosmetic Surgery (ABCS) tells us that "cosmetic surgery and plastic surgery are not the same thing." Meanwhile, the Canadian Society for Aesthetic Plastic Surgery reminds us that it is "the only professional organization in Canada dedicated to improved cosmetic surgery outcomes through education, research, and the maintenance of high surgical standards of clinical practice." That's not to exclude the Canadian Academy of Cosmetic Surgery, "founded out of the need to regroup physicians from the various surgical and medical disciplines whose special interest was anti-aging and cosmetic medicine." Almost any cosmetic clinic worth its salt employs some kind of laser, so the Canadian Laser Aesthetic Surgery Society is dedicated to excellence in cosmetic laser surgery. The Canadian Association of Aesthetic Medicine is clear however, that it is "the only national voice for aesthetic medicine in Canada."

I could go on and on. I've hardly touched on the U.S. boards, academies, societies and associations, to say nothing of the rest of the world. My point in mentioning a few is not to make light of fine professional organizations, but to underline that the closer you look at the field you're about to enter as a patient, the more there is to see.

The confusion between "plastic surgery" and "cosmetic surgery" illustrates my point. The ABCS defines plastic surgery as "a surgical specialty dedicated to reconstruction of facial and body defects due to birth disorders, trauma, burns, and disease. Plastic surgery is intended to correct dysfunctional areas of the body and is reconstructive in nature." The same organization defines cosmetic surgery procedures as enhancing a person's appearance toward some aesthetic ideal and notes that cosmetic medicine is practiced by "doctors from a variety of medical fields including dermatologists, facial plastic surgeons, general surgeons, gynecologists, oral and maxillofacial surgeons, ophthalmologists, otolaryngologists, plastic surgeons, as well as doctors from other fields."

Where practitioners are drawn from such a variety of

backgrounds and where there is not—and probably cannot be—a single authority, you're going to see overlapping claims and some friction. As much as a single group—plastic surgeons, say— would prefer to enjoy a monopoly, the simple fact is that there are other doctors equally capable of performing plastic procedures, and there are cosmetic procedures for which many plastic surgeons have little training. Successful cosmetic medicine requires a careful fitting of client to procedure, something the more traditional medical model of plastic surgery may not equip a doctor to do.

But it isn't my intention to criticize a profession or trumpet one over the other. In fact, all distinctions are washed away in a field where relentless change is the status quo. New procedures are constantly introduced and old skills become redundant. It's impossible that one institution, one set of criteria, one certification or one board will be the one solution for all time.

The subject of cosmetic surgery training often comes as a shock to people outside the field. As the ABCS writes, "there are currently no residency programs in the United States devoted exclusively to cosmetic surgery." There are none in Canada either. Doctors who wish to enter the field must get their training after they complete their residency. And you are right to wonder, training in what? A person may become proficient at removing moles with a laser or applying a chemical peel without having the slightest competency in liposuction. A surgeon may be able to remove your appendix but have no experience whatsoever with facelifts. And I don't want to leave you with the impression that anyone who takes it in mind to perform cosmetic procedures is as good as anyone else. The rigorous training and learning that lies behind every proper medical degree is an absolute prerequisite for even the most basic cosmetic procedures. If it's not a real doctor who performs the procedure in a clinic, it must be someone trained and supervised by a real doctor and even then only for limited procedures that do not require extensive medical experience. This is the starting line. Our discussion throughout this book is about what lies beyond that bare minimum.

How do you proceed? You don't have a single infallible source of information, so I must ask you now to look in the mirror. Looking back at you is not only a prospective cosmetic patient, but the ultimate source of information that must guide you to the right doctor. I haven't written this book to lecture and instruct. I've written it to elicit the best advice available from others in my field and to offer you tools I hope you'll apply to your own very personal situation, your place and time.

You're on your own, in other words, but I'm here to help you.

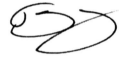

Barry Lycka M.D.

Contents

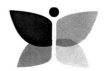

1 COSMETIC DOCTORS
The Best And The Rest

ur bodies are the vessels of our lives so it's not surprising we're all quite interested in the subject. Since ancient times humans have appreciated the healthy body—indeed, the Greeks seem almost to have worshipped it. And it was the Greeks too who advanced the study of medicine, that is, the restoration of health to the afflicted body. (I saw first-hand evidence of their exquisite knowledge 350 years before Christ at the temple of K'ombo—a temple built during the Greek Ptolemy era after Alexander the Great invaded Egypt.) These attitudes are firmly entrenched in modern times, when fitness and health are almost obsessions for many.

But one closely related area of body science stands somewhat alone: cosmetic medicine. The reason is perfectly simple: it hardly existed fifty years ago. No wonder our ideas about it are in a state of transition.

If you're reading this book, it's probably because you've become increasingly aware of the potential of cosmetic procedures and are starting to think about a cosmetic procedure for yourself. We sometimes refer to this growing awareness as "the disease of the Os"—as in "four-oh," "five-oh" or "six-oh." When people hit those decades, they begin to realize their limitations and they start worrying. They start saying, "Jeez, I don't feel like I'm fifty. I really feel like I'm maybe thirty." They look at these changes that come with age and ask, "Do I really want to live with them?" They say "I don't feel this way, I sure don't want to look this way." Of course if they do want to accept these changes, great: they can grow old gracefully. But if they don't, in this wonderful new age, they don't have to.

I'm willing to guess that you experience some apprehension when you think about the prospect of your own cosmetic procedure, however radical or minimal. I have heard and seen this thousands of times. I've written this book to help lessen that apprehension by placing more control in your hands. There are many many books that describe cosmetic procedures. I've recently written one myself: *SkinWorks: How to Restore and Keep Your Natural Beauty*. But my concern here is to help you in a practical way with the biggest decision of all: Who will perform the cosmetic work you're considering?

Is there a reason for fear? So it appears. It seems you can't pass the tabloid rack in your supermarket without seeing some cosmetic surgery disaster. Look at the celebrities who have experienced these disasters: Pricilla Presley (once gorgeous, now deformed), Heidi Fleiss (whom you can scarcely recognize) and Donda West, the mother of the famous rapper Kanye West, who paid the ultimate price for her attraction to cosmetic surgery—her life. Such rare catastrophes hardly ever happen and need not happen. For the vast majority of people seeking cosmetic procedures, the outcomes range from fantastic to not wholly satisfactory. In your own case, it's you who will determine the outcome through your choices.

Getting Cosmetic Surgery Right

Before we peel back the surface and look at the secrets to finding a doctor who can bring about your cosmetic surgery success, I'd like to take a closer look at some common misunderstandings about cosmetic science that naturally arise when a field advances so quickly. These misconceptions are subtly conveyed to us by our parents, the media and just folks we meet every day. They may be overtly communicated or lurk below the surface. Relatively recent television series such as *Sex and the City* or *Friends* might suggest one way of seeing cosmetic medicine. But for some of the important people in our lives—our parents perhaps—it might be more likely that the old Dick Van Dyke Show shaped their views and those were very different views indeed. (If you are unaware of the attitudes, look at an old show. Or read Dick Van Dyke's recently published autobiography). What was the attitude? A cosmetic procedure was something taboo, something hidden, never to be discussed except with your closest confidants. You got cosmetic surgery, hid away for months or years, then emerged from your treatment, much like a caterpillar morphing into a butterfly. Many patients tell me that their friends understand their interest

A cosmetic procedure was something taboo, something hidden, never to be discussed except with your closest confidants.

in cosmetic surgery but their mothers—or fathers—do not. We're witnessing a generational difference that's a consequence of rapid change. Perhaps most mothers of women now in their middle age harbour some of the beliefs about cosmetic surgery imbibed in the Dick Van Dyke era. Perhaps as a direct consequence they believe the subject should not be spoken of and that it's simply wrong to try and change the looks God gave you. Yet it's clear a younger generation feels differently. They feel they have the right to decide the way they look, and if something bothers them, they need not live with it.

What brought about this change? No doubt an important element was the discovery of Botox as a cosmetic agent. Botox transformed cosmetic surgery, took it out of the closet, made it the vogue thing to do. It became simple, safe, something you can do in minutes and have results that lasted months. You'd brag about it, even get it at a "Botox party." It became a lifestyle decision and

I suspect we haven't seen the last of the Botox breakthroughs. Meanwhile this new perspective is being transmitted to the older generation. Several times in the last few months I have had mothers visit me accompanied by their daughters—the daughter buying their mother a "thank you" present. Times really have changed.

The Myths

This generational divide has given rise to a number of myths about cosmetic procedures. Let's look at a few.

1.   *Cosmetic surgery only makes people feel better.*

Funny, one of the things our patients emphasize over and over is that cosmetic procedures first and foremost do make them feel better. But today it's understood that that's not the sole benefit. Cosmetic surgery has evolved dramatically

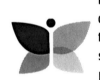

In the "old days" we just didn't have the treatments that could really make significant differences in people's lives.

in recent decades. In the "old days" we just didn't have the treatments that could really make significant differences in people's lives. Now we can help you lose inches, remove aging spots, lift your face (with and without surgery), get rid of stretch marks, remove wrinkles and much, much more. We can help you roll back the clock, reduce stress, and live a better, more successful, productive and healthy life.

Modern cosmetic medicine at its best actually does improve your looks but in a surprisingly subtle and natural way. You don't just feel better, you look better, and as a result, you live better.

2. Cosmetic surgery can be dangerous.

 $\mathcal{L}$ et me offer you an example to explain how this myth arose. I've been doing liposuction for twenty-five years. The very first case I saw was in 1986, during my residency. It was done under general anesthesia. The problem was that the medications that put the patient to sleep also dilated the blood vessels, causing bleeding—a lot of bleeding. The doctor had to use enormous cannulas to get into and out of the area being liposuctioned before the person would bleed to death. Also, for each litre of fluid taken out, two litres of packed cells had to be given to replace the fluid losses. More dangerously, bleeding caused clots to form that could move to the lungs, causing a pulmonary thrombo-embolism that could kill the patient. Even if something as catastrophic didn't occur, the large cannulas left a huge number of irregularities and recovery would take weeks if not months. No wonder people said that liposuction didn't work!

None of this is true today of liposuction. It's fast, safe, with predictable results and very little down time. Aided by lasers and power-assisted instruments, it is a marvelous treatment for the doctor and the patient. It has relatively few risks.

But how do we reconcile this with the highly publicized deaths that have occurred in cosmetic surgery? By recognizing that well-trained and experienced doctors dramatically decrease the risk of complications. That's what this book is about.

3. You should wait as long as possible.

 $\mathcal{S}$ ince cosmetic surgery used to be relatively dangerous and unpredictable, with the skill of the doctor being paramount, many doctors and patients did not feel the risks were worth it until there had been significant cosmetic decay. But during the 1980s a plethora of new, minimally invasive procedures evolved. Their hallmark was decreased risk and downtime.

Take, for example, Botox. The discovery that Botox relaxed the muscles that cause wrinkles associated with movement was serendipitous. Dr. Jean Carruthers, a Vancouver-based opthalmologist, was using it on a patient to treat an eye condition when her husband Alistair, a dermatologist, walked in. "What do you like best about Botox?" he asked. "It gets rid of my wrinkles," said the patient. So was the modern age of cosmetic surgery launched.

Botox works best early on in the wrinkling process. It can remove those "dynamic" wrinkles and act to prevent the formation of deeper wrinkles. The same is true of the now rapidly evolving filling agents. Used early on, they reverse and delay aging. Later in life, they have a different role: they are used to replace volume loss, one of the primary things that occur as we age. Lasers used to rejuvenate the skin work still differently. They repair the cells that support the foundation. Without fixing the skin tones and colour, it is virtually impossible to repair the deeper structural damage and this repair is more successful at an earlier stage.

Far from something we want to delay as long as possible, the application of cosmetic science has shifted towards early intervention.

Far from something we want to delay as long as possible, the application of cosmetic science has shifted towards early intervention. "Fix it fast so it will last" and "less is more" are the new mantras. Just like your car, your body needs ongoing maintenance. The longer you wait, the more difficult it is to repair the damage.

In one of my early books, I counseled cosmetic surgeons that fixing the skin is like a baseball game. More games are won by getting a player to first base, then to second and finally to third and home than by relying on home run hitters who strike out more often than not. Today, at my seminars, I tell audiences that modern cosmetic surgery is like modern math, where one plus one doesn't necessarily equal two; it sometimes equals three or five or ten. The combination of minor cosmetic procedures, started early, often creates a result greater than the sum of the smaller procedures.

4. One cosmetic doctor is just as good as another.

Does anyone believe this anymore? If it were true, I wouldn't be writing this book, would I? Even when surveying the best cosmetic doctors, it's important to know that doctors have various abilities and skills, just like athletes, leaders and generals. When you think about this, why would it be different in medicine? Some quarterbacks can throw the ball on a dime, others can read defenses well, others can run the ball. Sure, they're all great athletes, but if you were a general manager you'd need to choose the player with the skills for the job. Likewise, if I were looking to build a hockey team, I'd concentrate more on the Wayne Gretzkys and Mark Messiers than the Dave Semenkos. You win more games with top players who do what they love.

I love doing liposuction. I love every aspect of it and I love the patients who get it done. I can hardly sleep at night before a case, I'm so engaged. But when it comes to nose or breast jobs, it's a different story. My friend Dr. Gerry Goldberg, whom I spent a fair bit of time with in Tucson, loves lasers. But give him a facelift and he'd sooner take a rare day off. At this point in our careers, Gerry and I get enough of the type of cases we specialize in. We can leave other work to those with the appropriate calling. But many docs—"Jacks of all trades"—do whatever comes along because they have to, not because they want to. "Masters of all trades" such as my friend Charles Crutchfield of Minnesota are the exception, not the rule. Generally speaking, the physician's passion coupled with his or her ability, is what leads to successful outcomes.

From your perspective, it's caveat emptor: let the buyer beware. You must choose the doctor with the right set of skills for your needs—and the doctor you feel comfortable with. That's what this book is about.

5. *Having the right equipment is all a cosmetic doctor needs.*

*Y*eah right. Some laser companies would love to have the patient and the doctor believe this one. Of all the myths, it's perhaps the most dangerous. Medicine is still part art and part science, and the art component is the most difficult to quantify. Not every painter is a Rembrandt or a Monet. They can have the same brushes and paint but results, er, vary. The same can be said of cosmetic doctors and surgeons.

Many cosmetic doctors own or rent equipment but their training for their staff using that equipment is highly variable. And many laser companies feel it's per-

And many laser companies feel it's perfectly okay if doctors who have had only a few days training offer treatment on living patients.

fectly okay if doctors who have had only a few days training offer treatment on living patients, patients who would never knowingly consent if this was, say, an appendectomy.

The equipment itself also varies immensely in quality. This is particularly true in the case of laser hair removal. Some machines are under-powered to the point of being useless. Others are difficult to use. Consumers have been falsely led to believe that equipment quality is consistent and all they need do to be forever happy is find the cheapest treatment. Can any aesthetician do laser hair removal? Unfortunately not. I have seen many unhappy people in my office who went somewhere and did not get the results they thought they were going to get. I've seen many people actually scarred because they adopted this philosophy.

Like other conscientious cosmetic practitioners, I'm constantly investigating new equipment. I recently returned from Montreal, where I was checking out the newest model of a machine that helps remove fat without surgery or downtime. I actually looked into this technology years ago but it wasn't ready to use then. Now, it may have come of age—five years after my initial interest. In Montreal I visited the master, Dr. Arie Benchetrit, who has done more cases using this equipment than any other doctor. He also gets the best results. I brought one of my staff members with me and she underwent the treatment. But even if I buy this new machine, my staff will have to learn how to use it and there will be a learning curve. Far more than the equipment itself will determine our success.

6. *The wise shopper looks for the lowest price.*

*M*aybe when buying cars or shoes—but not always when paying for changes to your body. I'll guarantee that you've had the experience of buying a low-priced item only to be disappointed—who hasn't? In one of the conversations later in the book, my friend Charles Crutchfield, reminds me of the sign he remembers hanging in an old shoe repair shop in Minneapolis: "The bitterness of poor quality lasts much longer than the sweetness of low price."

Let's say we are talking about cars. How could the cheapest car be the best? If I offered to sell you a Lexus for $1000, wouldn't you wonder, "What's wrong with this car? A really good car should cost more than a clunker."

Warning: the price you see offered may not be for the procedure you want performed. I do a special type of liposuction known as Smart Laser ultrasound-assisted and power-assisted tumescent liposuction and very few practitioners do this advanced form, though many do liposuction of some kind and advertise the fact. Their prices are obviously different than mine.

And alas, the price you see offered may not be the price you pay. Quite often a low price is used to attract clientele, but when a full assessment is done, a much higher price is offered. Is this bait-and-switch advertising? You be the judge.

In the interests of improving the standards of my profession, I've dedicated my business to educating the public. The only way you can make an intelligent decision is to have all the facts you need. To that end, our clinic belongs to about two dozen organizations and I've been a founding member of Doctors for the Practice of Safe and Ethical Aesthetic Medicine, a group that believes firmly that "the patient comes first." We want our clientele to have the advantage the best cosmetic surgery procedures on the planet.

Make sure you get an exact price quote over the phone. Every doctor will give you one.

I wish you could but you can't. As in any cosmetic procedure, the prices differ drastically with the many variables. This is why no legitimate practitioner can give you a price on the phone. If you phoned your mechanic and told him that you had a terrible noise coming from the hood, then asked him for a quote, what do you suppose his response would be? We must see you, determine what is right for you and then determine exactly what you must do to achieve that. Then we'll give you a price. That's the only ethical way to do it.

If you phoned your mechanic and told him that you had a terrible noise coming from under the hood, then asked him for a quote, what do you suppose his response would be?

We must learn to live with imperfections.

*Y*ou know the old saying, "If God wanted us to fly, He'd have given us wings." But in fact God gave us something better: airplanes. The same is true of cosmetic surgery. As one of my patients said, "When God didn't get it right, He gave us cosmetic surgeons."

The Search Begins: What are Doctors Made of?

The biggest determinant of good cosmetic surgery is the choice of a cosmetic doctor and many people go about making this choice in the wrong way because they don't have the faintest idea how to do it. They Google or they look in the yellow pages or maybe they see the big glossy ads on the billboards or television; maybe they even go bargain hunting. But you can't really determine the quality of a cosmetic surgeon by the quality of an ad because an ad is meant to draw attention, not evaluate various claims. But through my now quite lengthy experience, I've found that the doctors who are at the top of this field—the ones at the cutting edge, so to speak—have different qualities, different traits, different habits, and different behaviors from the run-of-the-mill professional. Please allow me to showcase for you some of these characteristics.

7. *Curiosity*

The first trait you notice in the best cosmetic doctors is that they have an insatiable curiosity. They really want to know how things tick; they really want to get under the hood, so to speak. It's almost a hunger they have to fill.

I recently interviewed Dr. Nikolas Chugay, a well known cosmetic surgeon in the Beverly Hills and Long Beach area of Los Angeles http://www. drchugay.com/. Chugay was already doing breast implants but he also noticed that some people re- ally didn't like the way their butts were shaped. He was genuinely curious about whether he could help these people and he went on to become one of the first doctors to develop the buttock implant. I think of this procedure as a manifestation of Chugay's insatiable curiosity. He just couldn't rest until he'd figured out how to fix a problem that bothered a considerable number of his patients.

On another occasion Dr. Chugay heard about the "tongue

patch" from Dr. Luis Nader in Mexico. A tongue patch—about the size of a postage stamp and literally sewn on the top of the tongue—decreases appetite and helps with rapid weight loss, an interesting solution to some patients' weight problems. It intrigued Dr. Chugay to the point where, as he explains, he had to fly down to Mexico immediately. This was the time of the swine flu epidemic, so whereas a lot of people might be trying to sneak out of Mexico, he actually had to sneak into Mexico to learn this procedure. Back in Los Angeles, he began practicing the tongue patch approach and he has since helped a lot of people lose weight quickly. The press often refers to it incorrectly as the Chugay tongue patch.

I myself did the same with the threadlift. I heard about it in France several years ago and had to learn more. I flew to Mexico to learn this innovative technique. I subsequently did hundreds of cases before the company making the threads stopped during the great recession

Doctors such as Chugay—and I like to think I'm one of them—are re-creators and re-inventors. They may take the procedures they learn from other doctors but they make those procedures their own because they want the best of the best.

8.   Seekers of Greater Knowledge

This is a closely related quality. The best cosmetic surgeons are those who are in command of everything currently known about their area of specialty. They're constantly learning.

I started doing liposuction back in 1986 but the way I do liposuction now is a far cry from the way I did it in 1986. As I wrote earlier, back then the procedure could be dangerous because we had to put people under total anesthesia. In this state, two things could happen. First, patients would bleed a lot and so would require blood transfusions. With the emergence of AIDS and our greater understanding of hepatitis, we soon appreciated the dangers of these transfusions. Second, people put to sleep for a procedure are in danger of developing blood clots and clots can move to the heart or lung. Such clots are usually responsible for the rare cosmetic surgery deaths you'll read about in the newspaper.

But in 1989, my colleague Dr. Jeffrey Klein of San Juan Capistrano, California, developed a way to perform liposuction using local anesthesia. His technique is called tumescent liposuction and entails the removal of fat using only local anesthesia.

Now my patients may have liposuction done on a Thursday or a Friday and be back at work by Monday or Tuesday.

Since his discovery, we've all been doing it that way. And the innovation hasn't stopped. Lasers now melt the fat before we do any suctioning and new instruments such as the vibrating tools used in power-assisted liposuction dramatically reduce tissue trauma. Now my patients may have liposuction done on a Thursday or a Friday and be back at work by Monday or Tuesday, sore but able to continue their regular activities while their body responds to the surgery. Within one month, we're usually seeing phenomenal results.

I subsequently learned several techniques that compete with liposuction—more correctly called suction lipolysis. One of these is injection lipolysis—injecting chemicals into fat to help it disappear. I also learned cryolipolysis—an interesting technique known as CoolSculpting that removes fat by freezing it. And I've already mentioned ultrasonic lipolysis as done by Dr. Benchetrit. The field grows but an expert cosmetic surgeon keeps up with it, modifies it, enhances it.

This adopting and then enhancing is far more common than you might think. Dr. Woffles Wu, a plastic surgeon in Singapore, learned Botox a few decades ago much as I did. In a recent interview on *Inside Cosmetic*

Surgery Today on WebTalkRadio.net http://webtalkradio.net/ internet-talk-radio/2012/02/06/inside-cosmetic-surgery-to-day-%E2%80%93-botox-going-far-beyond-wrinkle-treatments-%E2%80%93-dr-barry-lycka-dr-woffles-wu/ he described to me his own progressive approach.

Botox was used first to diminish glabellar lines. Dr. Wu went on to use it for crows feet, with excellent results. He then began using it to lift the brow, often combining it with filling agents such as Restylane and Juvederm to get better results. He added in lasers and thread lifts and got results comparable to facelifts.

Then he did something that may be startling to some cosmetic doctors: he listened to his patients. He found that many of his female patients hated the "boxcar" jowly look that men liked and he began injecting the muscle in this area—the masseter—producing a more feminine look. He even injected the salivary glands in this area—the parotids—further enhancing the look.

His innovations did not end there. Finding that many of his patients did not want to look frozen by Botox, he began using small doses in the skin, not the muscle. This had the effect of beautifying the skin by decreasing the oil glands and large pores that can make the skin unattractive. He called these techniques MicroBotox and MesoBotox.

More recently, Dr. Wu began using Botox combined with intense pulsed light (IPL) therapy and cortisone injections—a treatment he calls triple therapy—to treat hypertrophic and keloidal scars and has achieved better results than traditional treatments. And finally, he has begun using Botox to prevent scar formation, especially in breast surgery.

9. *Excellence*

A third trait is the best cosmetic surgeons' hunger for excellence. They're just never satisfied with mediocrity. They're always looking for that edge. If something can make a little bit of difference, they want to try it, they want to go for it. They want to be the best in their profession and they're always looking at how they can be that best. This is such a noticeable feature within the profession, I started a MasterMind club for some of the most outstanding cosmetic surgeons on the planet. Several times a year, we come together to share our knowledge and learn from one another. We meet to discuss how we can become better.

10. *Sharing*

The best cosmetic surgeons love to share. They're not intimidated by other doctors and those who are the most sharing are often the best of the best. These same doctors also tend to share with others in their communi-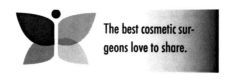ty by giving to charity and developing programs that go beyond their regular practice.

The best cosmetic surgeons love to share.

At our practice in Edmonton, we have several programs I'm proud of. We've found that many people who are gang members would love to get out of their gangs but they're virtual prisoners of their gang identity. Tattoos are a part of that identity and our clinic removes tattoos for free from people who are gang members. Liberated from these stigmas, many go on to become productive members of society. We realized that there are others whose tattoos can make them prisoners of an identity they'd rather leave behind: many prostitutes, for example, are tattooed by their pimps. We started a program to remove these tattoos without fee and we've had some amazing success stories. We had a visit recently from a lady whose tattoos we'd removed a few years earlier. She now has a little baby and is following a career as a social worker.

A number of years ago, we started the Victims of Spousal Abuse Program, whereby we gave victims of spousal abuse free reconstructive surgery, which is not normally covered by the healthcare system in any way, nor by any insurance plan. You will hear more about this a bit later when I talk to Sarah Burge, the "living Barbie doll."

When I'm doing a major seminar, I charge an attendance fee and that money goes to charity. For example, we're doing a seminar that charges a $25 contribution on behalf of the Canadian Skin Cancer Foundation, which I founded. The foundation's goal is "a world without skin cancer." We'd love to see the day when we never have to treat a skin cancer again. Every year we go to about seventy Alberta classrooms to educate hundreds and thousands of students about how to protect themselves from the sun, which is a major contributing factor for skin cancer. We are now expanding our program across the country and hope to soon go global.

11. Communication

When doctors successfully communicate with

> Cosmetic surgery is most effective when it's improving the lives of people who are not in crisis.

patients and uncover what's really bothering them, we can sometimes help in ways that are almost beyond belief.

A few years ago, I had a gentleman come in who wanted to get an eye lift done and I simply asked him why. He started crying and told me that his wife had died recently and that he was dealing with a lot of issues and was feeling ashamed of himself. I told him, "You really don't need to get your eye lift done right now. You really need to see a counselor and deal with the grief that you're going through." He came back to me several years later and he was so grateful that I'd been able to deal with the real problem, rather than something that he perceived to be the problem. Cosmetic surgery can be life altering for the good, but in this man's case, I questioned whether it was what he really needed. When people are going through breakups, divorces, bereavement, their emotional resources are needed elsewhere, not for cosmetic surgery. Cosmetic surgery is most effective when it's improving the lives of people who are not in crisis. But we must listen to our patients. That's communication.

12. Ethics

A great cosmetic surgeon is ethical and moral. He takes into account, above all, the needs and wants of his patients. As a bad joke has it: "Why did the plastic surgeon do a face lift? Because he had a mortgage payment due on his house in Newport Beach."

This may be a joke, but there are worrying occurrences in the real world. A few years ago, a Toronto cosmetic surgeon had a liposuction patient die after surgery. Ontario's College of Physicians and Surgeons found the doctor incompetent, and held that she'd failed to uphold the medical standard of practice in relation to her care of multiple cosmetic surgery patients. As a result this doctor had her certificate suspended for two years although she was allowed to assist in surgeries after that.

Earlier, I mentioned the death of Donda West, the mother of rapper Kanye West. The story is illustrative. On November 10, 2007, Donda West died of complications from cosmetic surgery involving abdominoplasty and breast augmentation. TMZ, a celebrity web site, reported that Beverly Hills plastic surgeon Andre Aboolian refused to do the surgery because Donda West had a health condition that placed her at risk for a heart attack. Aboolian referred her to an internist to investigate her cardiac issue. Donda never met with the doctor recommended by Aboolian and had the procedures performed by a third doctor, Jan Adams. West was 58 years old.

Certain unsafe doctors who do not or cannot act according to their patients' best interests should not be practicing.

You must choose a doctor who has, beyond anything else, your safety at heart. Cosmetic surgery is for the most part safe, but there are risks. Certain unsafe doctors who do not or cannot act according to their patients' best interests should not be practicing; certain unsafe patients should not have procedures done.

What causes doctors to behave in such different ways in the face of various challenges and temptations? Why does a world-class cosmetic doctor do what he does while another may fall short under the same circumstances?

Abraham Harold Maslow (1908–1970) was an American professor of psychology at Brandeis University, Brooklyn College, New School for Social Research and Columbia University. Maslow stressed the importance of doctors focusing on the positive qualities in people, as opposed to treating them as a 'bag of symptoms.' He argued that what compelled people (including doctors) to act in a certain way were needs, which he arranged in a hierarchy, now commonly referred to as Maslow's Hierarchy of Needs.

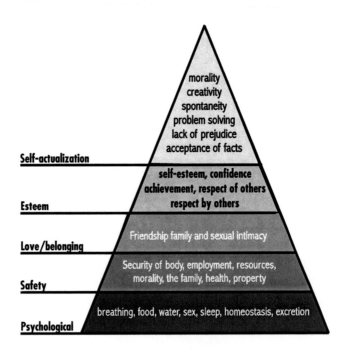

Like everyone else, some doctors are motivated to make money to "pay the bills" and we must position them near the bottom of the pyramid. These are the doctors who "sell" patients procedures they might not want or need. Others will stick to traditional thinking in all circumstances because they fear sanction by their colleagues. They're a little higher up. Still others are motivated by belonging or esteem needs. But the best cosmetic doctors are motivated by self-actualization: They do what's right for their patients because it's the right thing to do. When tools are not at hand, they invent them.

13. Free Thinking

As Maslow suggests, the best doctors are free thinkers who do not limit themselves to the ideas as they exist today. My former chairman in the Department of Dermatology at the University of Minnesota, Peter Lynch, was a man of this type. In the first lecture he gave to our class as residents he drew a square on a blackboard. He surrounded it by another square, then another, then another. In the first square he wrote "knowledge in textbooks." In the second he wrote "knowledge in journals." In the third he wrote "knowledge in seminars and lectures" and in the last "knowledge in the universe."

A first-class doctor doesn't only think outside the box, he creates a new box.

He turned to us.

> Doctor, as residents you will be required to learn the content of textbooks and journals. This is your life blood and it's what you'll be tested on. But be very aware that this is only a trifling part of the knowledge that is out there. At seminars and lectures, you'll learn far more. It hasn't been written yet. But be very aware that this is not the extent of knowledge. There is far more in the universe. It just that nobody's 'thunk' of it yet.

A first-class doctor doesn't only think outside the box, he creates a new box. Take, for example my friend Haines Ely. He is probably the most unconventional doctor on the planet. He is always thinking of new and better ways to improve his treatments.

An example. Haines was a patient for a surgical procedure. Like many doctors, he discharged himself from hospital too early. On his way home, he began to bleed profusely. Not wanting to embarrass himself by admitting he had done the wrong thing by leaving the hospital, he began to think. He thought back to the time he was a resident in internal medicine and doing a hematology rotation. (All doctors must spend time in different areas of medicine. The theory is that it'll make you a better doctor.) His professor had remarked off-hand how certain people have a biochemical problem that prevents them from metabolizing fat properly. "Isn't it funny how fatty blood doesn't bleed?" he's asked. A light turned on in Haine's brain. He stopped at a corner store and bought a Haagen Dazs ice cream bar. These things have huge amounts of fat in them, so much that even healthy people will have "fatty blood."

In less than twenty minutes, he stopped bleeding.

We see many patients who are on anti-coagulants to help prevent heart attacks and strokes. The downside is they also cause these people to bleed when they have surgery done. We often can't stop these medications for surgery. At one point I noticed when I was doing a cancer surgery that we hadn't had a bleed in quite awhile. "Unusual," I thought out loud. My nurse laughed.

"What did you do" I asked.

"Ice cream before surgery," she said. "I reasoned that if it stopped bleeding after surgery, bleeding might be prevented if we gave it before."

Brilliant—but it didn't stop there. If ice cream could prevent bleeding, could it prevent bruising? A bruise is a bleed that occurs within the tissue. We now give our patients ice cream before any surgery, any Botox or fillers and we find it decreases bruising markedly.

Such ideas that do not occur in books, journals or seminars but certainly they exist in "the universe" and we sometimes trip over them through good fortune and free thinking. A wise cosmetic doctor is guided by both.

14. Mastermind

We touched on this briefly but I must elaborate. The concept of the MasterMind group was formally introduced by Napoleon Hill in the early 1900s. In his classic, *Think And Grow Rich,* he wrote this about the Mastermind principle:

> [It is] the coordination of knowledge and effort of two or more people, who work toward a definite purpose, in the spirit of harmony....No two minds ever come together without thereby creating a third, invisible intangible force, which may be likened to a third mind.

In a MasterMind group, the agenda belongs to the group, and each person's participation is key. Their peers give them feedback, help them brainstorm new possibilities, and set up accountability structures that keep them focused and on track. By creating a MasterMind group, you create a community of supportive colleagues who will brainstorm together to move the group to new heights, allowing them to gain tremendous insights that can improve their business and personal lives. A MasterMind group is like having a objective board of directors. Members surround themselves with high functioning and like-thinking individuals. I was introduced to the MasterMind concept by Dan Kennedy, a businessman known as "the millionaire maker" who was also a professor of harsh reality. My life has never been the same since. He showed me the benefit of MasterMind clubs and I began running these for doctors as a result. Having gone through dozens of MasterMind encounters, I must tell you that this powerful experience—sharing with and learning from one's peers—differentiates the best doctors from the rest.

15. Intelligence

As a group, the best cosmetic doctors are among the brightest doctors I've met. Many, I'd say, could have been anything they wanted to be: nuclear physicists, heads of corporations, leaders of governments. They chose cosmetic surgery because it was their passion.

16. Integrity

Warren Buffett, one of the richest men in the world, once said that to be successful in any business you must be intelligent, goal-driven and have extreme integrity. Of these traits, integrity is the most important, because without it the other two traits will ultimately get you in trouble.

This is true of the best cosmetic doctors. They walk the walk and talk the talk. They embody integrity in everything they do. In the next chapter, Charles Crutchfield recounts how he avoided the "false Botox" scandal. Some years ago Charles went to a conference and sat next to the vice president of a company making a new form of Botox. He was almost convinced to use it but his moral compass pointed away. His patients' safety came first.

This "Botox" came from outside the United States and was imported into Arizona. It was Botulinum toxin, like true Botox, but the quality was dubious and the risk of using it turned out to be terrifying. The scandal broke when a doctor in Florida injected his wife and she became paralyzed and had to be put on a respirator to sustain her life. The regulatory officials started investigating and found other doctors were giving this false Botox to their patients. Many simply adjusted the dosage to stop the side effects.

The Qualities: A Summary

Curiosity, excellence, knowledge, "MasterMind" guidance, integrity, sharing, ethics, free thinking and communication;

these are the signs of a top cosmetic doctor. These are the sinews of their character.

I was once running a conference in Las Vegas with a number of doctors and we lost one of our number after dinner. He just vanished. Knowing that "what goes on in Vegas" can sometimes stay in Vegas, the rest of us set off to look for him in places of poor repute. In the end, however, we found him in the wee hours at a live music venue. He had cornered some professional musicians and had engaged them in a discussion, pumping them for a better understanding of their music. Here you could see all the factors rolled into one simple situation, factors that make the difference between the best cosmetic surgeons and the rest.

But all this amounts to my opinions and observations. I decided that a better way to provide an overview of my profession was to sit down with fellow professionals—some but not all of those I regard as the best—and let them talk. What follows in the next chapter is an account of those conversations.

2 CONVERSATIONS WITH THE BEST

Those who know me well know me to have strong ideas about what makes a first-class cosmetic doctor. I like to think that my own practice embodies many of these ideas because I've spent years trying to achieve that excellence. But when I set out to write this book, an early goal was to learn what other professionals believed. What informed their practices? What principles did they pursue?

I contacted Dr. Jeff Riopelle of San Ramon, California, Dr. Charles Crutchfield of Minneapolis, Minnesota, Dr. Scott MacKenzie of Corner Brook, Newfoundland, Dr. Daryl Hoffman of Palo Alto, California, Dr. Ron Moy of Los Angeles, and Dr. Steven Schlosser of Boulder, Colorado. I didn't pick these people at random. Each of them enjoys a sterling reputation and the respect of colleagues. They were the sort of doctors that, were a loved one of mine to seek cosmetic work, I wouldn't hesitate to recommend. As you read through our discussions, you're going to see how, yes, they sometimes disagree: these are people who think for themselves. But you'll also notice how certain themes reoccur, not once but several times. I haven't edited out these repetitions because they serve to highlight certain guiding principles, many of which I share.

Please note, not everyone on this list will be on television, in magazines, or elsewhere visible. Some like Scott MacKenzie quietly do their jobs. Others like me are in the news all the time.

Jeff Riopelle: The Good Listener

*M*y discussion with Jeff Riopelle brought out a great deal about how cosmetic practitioners find their way into this relatively new field and acquired the skills that make them the outstanding physicians they are.

Jeff is a family doctor in the San Ramon, California area. http://www.laseradvantage-medispa.com/ You might, at first blush, wonder how a family doctor can or should be a cosmetic surgeon. Let me explain. Dr. Riopelle's original interest was conventional surgery and his residency had been heavy on surgery. Indeed, Jeff still regularly "assists" in cardiac surgery in the operating room.

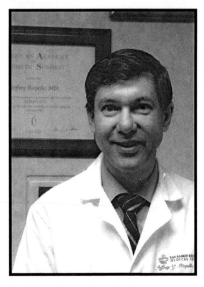

Jeff Riopelle is a family doctor in the San Ramon, California area, whose reputation as a compassionate physician had more to do with his cosmetic career than did his surgical training.

You might think that surgeons, with their orientation to hand/eye skills and their knowledge of what you can and can't do with human tissue, might be well equipped as cosmetic practitioners. But when I spoke to Jeff, he wanted to m   t surgical residents are taught few techniques that are applicable to modern cosmetic medicine. Rather, it was patients' questions about cosmetic procedures that were the spur to his interest. People were asking about Botox and liposuction and lasers. They'd heard about these things in the media and wanted to know more. There were few doctors who could answer their questions. And as Jeff gradually evolved his cosmetic practice, it was his work as a general practitioner that proved a major contributor to his success.

Indeed, I recently spent three days with 75 residents in dermatology from the leading medical schools in North America teaching them at a cosmetic congress in Las Vegas. I asked them, "How many have been taught anything about Botox or fillers?' I was surprised to find out how few had. I thought this was a thing of the past. When I was a resident quite a few moons ago, I was chastised by my chairman for even think-ing about these topics. But now, in the new millenni-um, I was certain times had changed. Apparently not.

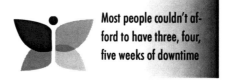

Most people couldn't af-ford to have three, four, five weeks of downtime

"Patients were looking for a good compassionate physician," Jeff said. "They were look-ing for someone who was a good listener and could take their needs and translate those needs into what they're looking for cosmetically."

In other words, it was his attention to his patients more than his interest in surgery that drew him forward and drew patients to him. He was a talented guy, but he understood that talent without compassion doesn't mean too much.

As he developed his cosmetic surgery skills, he became increas-ingly aware that what his patients wanted was no downtime or minimal downtime.

"Most people couldn't afford to have three, four, five weeks of downtime—as had often been the norm with cosmetic proce-dures. They were looking for doctors who'd trained in the most up-to-date, short-downtime procedures. I'd trained under some of the best physicians in the United States and Canada to learn the touch of that kind of cosmetic procedure."

In the course of his development, Jeff discovered something that all cosmetic practitioners come to understand: A body of medical opinion holds that you have to have a plastic surgery background to really be a competent cosmetic doctor. This opinion is strongest among some classic plastic surgeons, who naturally want to defend their turf, though please note that I know several who do not stick to this dictum. But these specialized plastic surgeons did their residence training in many areas other than just cosmetic surgery. In fact, they don't have nearly as much specific cosmetic training as people might think. A whole year of their training is in general surgery, operating on the bowel or the gallbladder—areas of expertise that really don't have anything to do with cosmetic surgery. And an important part of plastic surgery training is in the treatment of burn victims, wounds, hand injuries and doing tendon repairs. These skills too are highly tangential to cosmetic procedures. Sure, some of the manual treatment techniques are transferrable, but not all.

So I asked Jeff, what are the procedures that a successful and popular cosmetic surgeon performs today?

"As I say, we specialize in minimally invasive, low-downtime procedures, so our biggest areas are Smart Lipo and laser lipo, which we call Smart Lipo Ultra. We do pretty much every area of the body and it's all done under local "tumescent" anesthesia. We also do a lot of other minimal-downtime procedures on the face: Thermage for skin tightening, the thread lift, which is minimally invasive lifting of the skin, and the plasma laser, which is another minimally invasive resurfacing procedure of the skin. We do a variety of vein procedures, everything from minor spider veins to the more severely damaged veins that used to be removed surgically but that now can be removed with a laser."

But as he was describing these, one thought was foremost in my mind.

"You really didn't learn any of these procedures in your residency, did you, Jeff?"

"Not specifically, no."

Nor did I. And for most doctors that's true. The fact is, these procedures were in their infancy or non-existent when Jeff was doing his residency. Many doctors have had to learn their procedures outside of their residency. The way I practice medicine now is not the way I practiced it five years ago or the way I practiced it ten years ago. And tomorrow, it'll be far different. "It's where the puck is going to be, not where the puck is," said the greatest hockey player of all time, Wayne Gretzky.

"Virtually none of what I do today was even available when I was in residency training. The half-life of medical knowledge is supposedly about seven years, so every seven years half of what we used to do is no longer The half-life of medical knowledge is supposedly about seven years, so every seven years half of what we used to do is no longer done done or is no longer felt to be correct. So we always have to be updating ourselves and constantly improving and striving to attain the best that's available now."

In fact, so accelerated is the advancement of medical techniques, the half-life of knowledge might be five years by now—or even three and a half years. What used to be a gold standard ten years ago is no longer a gold standard. That's why the good physicians are people who really love to learn new things, the ones like Jeff Riopelle who love adapting to new procedures and integrating the newest into their practices.

"That's actually one of the reasons I went into cosmetic surgery—because it's so rapidly changing, it allows us to really be on the cutting edge all the time."

The Machines

*I*f you've paid the slightest attention to cosmetic surgery, you'll know that procedures employing a wide variety of sophisticated devices are on offer to the public. What you may not know is that these devices pose an ongoing challenge for cosmetic clinicians.

Jeff Riopelle told me how he was one of the lead experimenters trying out a new piece of equipment, a machine that was supposed to get rid of fat without any surgery. He then reported to his group that he had to struggle sometimes to determine which was the "pre" and which was the "post"—in other words, whether the equipment had made any difference at all. Charitably described, the results were so subtle that they were almost non-existent. Skeptical surgeons had to wonder whether the improvements existed in the investigators' minds and in the patients' minds, rather than in reality.

The truth is that companies spend big dollars developing such equipment, so they have a huge motivation to get it out onto the market. But when people start paying for it, it may come out at last that it doesn't work. As Jeff says, the only defense a patient has against such ineffective treatments is to find a physician who is well respected, who is honest with them and who doesn't try to sell them treatments that don't work well—in other words, a physician who never puts his interests ahead of his patients' interests. Sadly, many physicians are sold equipment that doesn't really work and they're then tempted to foist it on patients because it has to be paid for.

My own experience had been to go to conferences and find people on the podium who were literally prostituting themselves, talking about laser systems that had never worked once in my office. I met doctors who were being paid by companies—they were shills, really—up there talking about procedures that didn't make sense. And I found that many of these doctors wouldn't share whatever they'd discovered that did work. This whole culture of cosmetic medicine seemed broken and I decided to fix it in my own way. I turned to the Mastermind concept, which is built around professionals forming informal associations that allow them to learn and share in confidence. I assembled a group of like-minded doctors, doctors who loved to share.

Jeff too joined my MasterMind group.

"It was by far the best learining medical environment I'd ever been in," he confirmed. "People were open to one another and willing to share ideas, willing to share new experiences, willing to say, 'I know a lot about that particular procedure and it doesn't work.'

"When I first began to offer laser surgery, I was at the mercy of salespeople. A couple of the lasers I bought did virtually nothing. But once I joined the MasterMind group, there was always someone who had personal expertise in that particular piece of equipment and could tell me how well it worked—or not. Even today, our group of eight, ten, twelve cosmetic surgeons—specialists in our various areas of cosmetic surgery—we exchange ideas and basically teach one another. Believe me, I've been saved numerous times from buying new pieces of equipment that were the newest, the latest and the greatest but that didn't work that well."

Like Jeff, I too had found that laser salesman were often too ready to tell me how a laser would shine my shoes, recite Shakespeare and improve my sex life. Lasers are wonderful machines when they work properly but unfortunately the vast majority of them are more hype than reality. It's not the equipment that makes the process, it's the doctor that makes the process.

"So there's a rule for patients," Jeff says. "Look for a physician who belongs to something like a Mastermind group—a peer group that exchanges ideas."

Yes, do that, and remember that even board certification may not mean everything. What's more important than any official recognition is that a doctor be willing to learn a new procedure and learn it well.

Jeff told me that when he started learning liposuction, the standard of care—that is, the training necessary to be a liposuction physician—was simply taking a two-day training course and beginning to bill for your service. Nothing required you to attend other practices in order to learn from other doctors. No one required you to take the best from all those doctors and then amalgamate it into your own practice. These were things you did on your own initiative.

"I took many courses before I knew I was ready to start performing a procedure on regular patients," he told me. "I tried it on many family members and friends, honing my skills. Finally I would say, "Okay, I'm ready to do this for a member of the public."

Patient, Help Thyself

*P*atients too have a responsibility. To start with, they can avoid doing dumb things when they're looking for a cosmetic doctor.

"Right," Jeff said. "One of the things patients can avoid is going to those rating sites on the Internet. Surely it's obvious that anybody can put anything on them. A jealous colleague, for example can write a bad review about

One of the things patients can avoid is going to those rating sites on the Internet.

somebody and from the patient's standpoint, there's no way to determine whether the damning comment was even posted by a patient who had visited the doctor in question."

Anonymity may be valuable in the polling booth but Jeff feels it can be invidious in the assessment of a professional. One site, Ratemds.com, tends to carry only negative comments. How could every doctor be bad? The Internet can be the most amazing resource and like the best library, it can be full of great books and great journals. Unfortunately

they're right next to the garbage and sometimes you can't be sure which is which.

"But people naturally turn to the Internet," Jeff says. "I feel they can learn the most by studying a physician's website and asking themselves, 'Is this doctor someone who's trying to teach me on this website? Is he trying to explain procedures to me? Does he offer instructional videos?' These are the kinds of things that can allow a patient to assess whether she or he could relate well to that physician. My mom was a teacher and my dad was a private in-

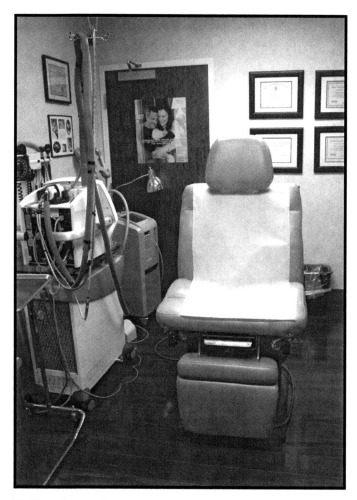

The Riopelle procedure room is well equipped but without flash, as befits a physician whose practice has grown from a base in family medicine. Those are his credentials on the back wall. Make sure your doctor has the equivalents.

vestigator. I feel I inherited the teaching impulse from my mom and the investigator from my dad. To me, the best physicians are actually teachers who love to share their information and their knowledge.

I suggest that another mistake some patients make when shopping for a cosmetic surgeon is to make their decision on the basis of price. Such people want good cosmetic surgery—but cheap.

"That's a big mistake," Jeff agrees, "because we're talking about a patient's body. Obviously quality must inform the decision before price."

That's certainly not what I'd want....I'd want good cosmetic surgery, not cheap cosmetic surgery.

We learn this from experience since all of us from time to time have purchased something on account of it being very cheap, only to be disappointed. Paying an exorbitant amount for goods and services is not the solution either; rather, in the market for any given good or service, we expect to pay a reasonable amount for a good product. Often, when I visit places like San Francisco and open up a local magazine, I see ads that offer cosmetic surgery at what they claim to be the lowest price on the planet. And I shake my head and say, "That's certainly not what I'd want if I was looking for cosmetic surgery." I'd shun such offers because, first and foremost, I'd want good cosmetic surgery, not cheap cosmetic surgery.

Finally, we turned to the subject of community service. As I've said elsewhere, a doctor's willingness to give back to the larger society is to me an important indicator of attitude. It didn't come as a surprise that Jeff Riopelle was actively engaged in charity work and the community outside his own immediate circle. He's been a basketball and little league coach and devoted his time to a Halloween candy "buy-back" program that sponsors school projects and sends the candy to U.S. troops overseas. As an extension of his work, he gives frequent seminars but donates a portion of the seminar fees to charitable causes. In the course of all these activities, he either acts as a teacher himself or has regular contact with teachers he admires. This is yet another important indicator of the quality and character of the cosmetic surgeon you're looking for: A good doctor is a teacher by nature, not just a skilled handler of instruments.

The Foundations of Happiness

I asked Jeff what gave him the greatest satisfaction. He laughed.

"Well, that's difficult," he said. "On a personal level, my wife Donna and my four children, all of whom are perfect 4.0 students and all of whom I've coached either in basketball or baseball.

"In my practice, I think I relate well to my patients. I have been told that I'm a great listener. I try to understand patients' needs and desires and then create the optimal treatments for them.

"I also take satisfaction in being innovative. I was among the first doctors to combine IPL (intense pulsed light) with Laser Genesis before a major company, Cutera, came out with it as a single unit. I was also among the first doctors to do fat transfers to the buttocks as part of the Brazilian Butt Lift, and among the first in the U.S. to perform the Vampire facelift. I invented the RioLift (the three-dimensional facial rejuvenation), and was among the first in the U.S. to learn stem cell processing of fat."

There is no doubt that Jeff Riopelle is "ahead of the curve." He has been sought out as a research consultant by such major names as Solta (thermage) and Zeltiq (Cool Sculpting) and selected to TopDocAmerica the last two years in succession.

Charles Crutchfield: The Balanced Professional

*C*harles Crutchfield's credentials read like a list of accomplishments that might belong to a Nobel prize winner. He works in the greater Minneapolis area but sees patients from across the United States and from Europe and South America. This is something he and I have in common. There are cosmetic doctors in other parts of the world that do cosmetic surgery but we're honoured and thrilled when patients come from far away to see us.

Unlike Jeff Riopelle but like myself, Charles had been trained in classic dermatology. He joined a group of twelve other dermatologists in the early 1990s just as the new field of cosmetic dermatology was taking off. At that point, he was the only one of the group who had done any cosmetic work—Botox and fillers and lasers—so he became the resident expert in these areas. As his cosmetic practice has grown, however,

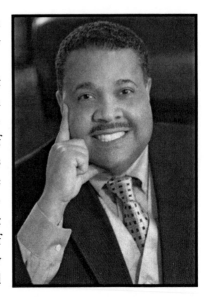

Dr. Charles Crutchfield is one of the leading cosmetic dermatologists in North America.

he has remained active as a medical dermatologist specializing in pediatric and geriatric dermatology. This balancing of cosmetic medicine with other aspects of medical practice is a characteristic I often see in the better cosmetic practitioners. In fact, it is something you should watch out for and score extra points for in your search for the best cosmetic surgeon. Physicians with balanced practices are more likely to be those who want to learn and serve. And from a practical perspective, the balanced practice broadens the scope of your physician's experienced-based knowledge.

When I considered all the many doctors doing cosmetic procedures in the Minneapolis area, I wondered why a particular patient might choose Charles Crutchfield. He thought about it for a moment.

"Well, it's true that when patients come to our office, they're inclined to feel comfortable. But we also make a serious effort to explain to them that experience counts and quality matters.

About six months ago, I got a call from a newspaper writer in Minneapolis. He said 'Hey, listen, I'm doing an article. How much do you charge for a unit of Botox?' I said, 'What's your article about?' He said, 'We're calling all of the offices and we're going to list everybody. What do you charge for Botox per unit?'

"I had to educate him. 'It's not really what is the cost per unit of Botox,' I said. 'The question you should be asking is, what value do patients get when they come in for a Botox treatment?'

"Unfortunately, there are doctors who actually will charge for Botox treatment by the unit and then they use far too many units and so the price goes up for the pa-

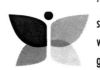

'The question you should be asking is, what value do patients get when they come in for a Botox treatment?'

tient. Or they'll hire an assistant who took a course in Las Vegas a month ago, practicing injections on tomatoes. These services may cost several dollars a unit less but they're not based on the same experience.

"I had a patient come in the other day and she was very upset. She said 'One of my friends gave me a certificate for a cosmetic treatment at another office and I went there and they didn't have a physician. They just had a nurse and the nurse did the treatment but the treatment didn't work out well. So I got this free treatment. And I have to tell you, it was worth every penny.'"

Every time I personally have been tempted to try and match a price, I've had to cut corners in some way. Since I'll never, ever cut quality, that unfortunately means my service comes at a slightly higher price. As Charles told me, "In our clinic we stand behind a treatment completely. If a patient isn't happy, we do whatever's necessary at no charge. Our goal is to make the patients happy because we plan on being there for a long time. But it's hard to live up to those standards if you're working on a cut-rate basis."

The fact is, if a cosmetic clinic is getting a lot of bargain shoppers, the clinic has to be doing a huge volume practice. They have to push those numbers to the max in order to earn a decent profit. For patients, this means a watered down experience to the point where it's really not a good experience. As I was writing this, I had a lady come in who'd had someone inject some filling substance into her lips. She was a bit dissatisfied because the result was uneven. I had to tell her I couldn't be certain what filling substance had been used but I hoped it was a temporary one because those lumps might otherwise be permanent. She was shocked to hear that. I offered to help, to get her

I had to tell her I couldn't be certain what filling substance had been used but I hoped it was a temporary one because those lumps might otherwise be permanent.

records and see what I could do but unfortunately she might be left with a blemish or worse.

Charles nodded. "When you're getting any cosmetic treatment, the important thing is not what's in the syringe but who's on the other end of it. When I was in medical school, I used to get my shoes fixed at an old shoe repair shop in the back of a house. They had a little thing hanging on the wall. It read: The bitterness of poor quality lasts much longer than the sweetness of low price.

Reputations spread through word of mouth and referrals from friends are everyone's best guide. But if you can't access that sort of personal referral, remember that most cosmetic clinicians advertise and maintain informative websites. Study those websites as though they were people and decide who you like and who you don't. Then—and this is a key point—go to the office. Make sure you feel comfortable with the set up there, and with the support staff. Then ask the doctor some questions. Charles had several suggestions for questions that everyone should ask.

"First," he asked, "what happens if you undergo a treatment and have an unwanted side effect or a complication? I had a patient who came in yesterday and she had gone to one of those mall spots supposedly staffed by a physician. The laser settings were wrong and she was scarred as a result. A terrible outcome. She asked to see the doctor and they said, 'He's not here.' She demanded to know when he would be there. 'He's going to come in next month,' they told her. She went back three times and never did see the physician.

"If you have a side effect, are you going to be seen by somebody who knows how to handle side effects? Our dermatology surgery mentor at the University of Minnesota, Dr. Zachary, would always call us in when he had a side effect or an unwanted result. He would get more excited about teaching us from these problems than about a really excellent result. To be a great physician, he'd say, you have to be able to handle complications. There's often more art than science involved because everybody heals differently and responds differently. You know this, Barry. We so often have to change the procedure to meet the patient."

Attention to our patients is the key. A good doctor looks at the whole picture, not just a little part of it. And a good doctor looks at it over and over again, constantly re-evaluating. Rosacea for example is often treated today with lasers. But rosacea is much more of a disease than a simple laser can handle. A good doctor may also treat it with antibiotics, with special creams, and by prescribing avoidance of things that might be precipitating the erythema (redness). As Charles says, clinicians who don't have training in skin care can buy a laser and set up shop and treat the redness but they may not treat the multiplicity of other factors that play into the disease.

Jeff Riopelle and I had spoken about the rapidly evolving state of medical knowledge. I wanted to hear what Charles had to say on the same subject.

"Is the way you practice medicine now the same as you practiced it maybe five years ago?" I asked.

"No. I think I reinvent myself every five years. The basics remain but you're constantly improving and getting better. A good doctor is always looking to develop that little edge for his patient. I trained at the Mayo Clinic and they used to say, 'First and foremost, do what is best for the patient and everything else will follow.'"

Unfortunately, not every doctor does that. Before thinking of their patients, some doctors are thinking of their economic well being or their vacations. And Charles reminds me that insurance companies and third party payers can exacerbate the situation by making increasingly tough demands on doctors, demands that may be related inversely to the quality of care.

"I'm actually getting letters from a lot of the insurance companies," he told me. "They're looking at how many generic

"One of the biggest mistakes patients can make," Charles says, "is failing to ask questions...."

medicines I've written that year and telling me that their goal for next year is for me to get it up to such and such a percent. They're not thinking about what's best for the patient. They're trying to get what's best for their bottom line."

I have to agree. I shock many patients when I express the opinion that generic medications are sometimes not as good as the gold standard medications. For example, I've observed hyper-pigmentation (increased darkening of the skin) with a certain medication, but never with the brand name product, only with the generic version. This observation is based on my patient records over a period of fifteen years. Who knows why this should be so? It could be something trivial in the processing cycle since a significant part of the effectiveness of many dermatological agents is based on the vehicle and its ability to penetrate the skin. But whatever the explanation, the problem is real enough that I resist the pressures to switch to the generic product.

"One of the biggest mistakes patients can make," Charles says, "is failing to ask questions. Ask the physician how long he or she has been providing these treatments. Ask for 'before and after' pictures of patients they've treated. Don't just ask if they're board certified in either dermatology or plastic surgery or ophthalmology or other related specialties. Simply ask about their experience. Ask where they got their training. Ask how many patients they've treated with your particular condition. Ask if they're doing any teaching or work with residents or medical students, because a good doctor wants to share knowledge. Ask what charities they're involved in because a good doctor is thinking about others."

A good cosmetic doctor, in other words, has to be a well-rounded, balanced individual. A good doctor will never take offense at such questions.

"And if you should go to a medical spa or clinic," Charles adds, "check out the medical director, the physician. Does he or she actually see patients and treat patients or is the doctor just a name that allows the spa to operate? Can you see her or him for a consultation?"

As a possible patient of a given doctor or clinic, you must act to some degree as your own detective. Watch for tell-tale signs of caring, aesthetic interests and thoroughness. Even cosmetic physicians should take a basic medical history because they must understand what is going on with the whole patient. Before I even see patients, my staff has them fill out a form telling me all the things that are going on with them. I can't make clinical decisions on cosmetic issues unless I know patients have a good heart and good lungs, whether they smoke (unfortunately, people don't heal as well when they smoke a lot) and what's currently going on in their lives (since people who are really stressed out don't heal well either).

Our conversation then turned to the anonymous Internet sites that "rate" doctors. Charles, like Jeff Riopelle and myself, condemned the anonymity of these listings. The site operators are totally absolved of responsibility because they are treated in law as bulletin boards. You can't sue a bulletin board.

Charles sighs. "I had a colleague who was going through a nasty divorce and his ex-wife just killed him on these sites. She went in and left all kinds of terrible messages about hurting babies and much more. But readers wouldn't know these comments were being left by a spouse in a divorce battle. They'd assume they were the work of a patient. I myself had a couple of negative reports put on me a couple of years ago that claimed I gave medication to a patient that was harmful to a baby. I looked at my records and I hadn't treated anyone pregnant around that time. Two years later, about a month ago, I get a call from a guy who told me that the negative comments had been put up by an employee who we'd let go some time before and she was having all kinds of problems and anger. And what about jealous competitors? What's to stop them from blackening a well-known rival's reputation? You don't know. It's anonymous."

Another Internet phenomenon are the sites that sell doctor's advice. A no-name doctor will give you advice on your acne for $49.99.

"All you need is a credit card," Charles says. "And sadly a lot of third party payers and insurance companies are actually experimenting with this level of medicine. They have a nurse practitioner on call 24 hours. You pay your $49 and she'll give you a prescription for hydrocortisone for your rash. You get what you pay for.

"The truth is, there are two very reliable sources of information. First, physicians in the community know who the other good physicians are because they refer patients to one another. Patients come back and report good results. The physicians know what's what. Second, your friends. These are the people who've had procedures done. They've been there. You can trust them. You don't want to go on a website and read some crazy anonymous verbiage. Talk to your friends and relatives and physicians. That will give you at least a good start on finding a quality cosmetic specialist.

"And bear in mind that, as a patient, it's your right to feel very comfortable. You don't want to feel like you are being pressured or rushed into doing anything."

Indeed, a patient should never feel pressured. They should never feel sold. They should never feel that they are being handled in a certain way. But at the same time they should have all their questions answered. Patients should go into a prospective doctor's office with their antennae up, feeling things out and observing as they go. Remember, how you're treated by that office before a procedure is the same way you're going to be treated after a procedure. And if something goes wrong, that's what matters.

Charles Crutchfield and I ended our discussion with the subject of patient safety. He recalled the false Botox scandal.

> Patients should go into a prospective doctor's office with their antenna up, feeling things out and observing as they go.

"I went to a medical conference some years ago. They were talking about this new "Botox" that was half the price of regular Botox. I followed it carefully but didn't buy it. Then one day I got a call from the Feds and they were asking if we knew about any fake Botox being sold in the area because they thought there was a shipment coming from China, something called Chinatox. Some of the people who'd been given this stuff had almost died.

"'I don't think it's Chinatox,' I told them. 'You better look at this place right down here in Arizona.' I got subpoenaed as a government witness. This product had very poor quality control and we were able to shut the whole thing down and help make Botox safe for everyone else."

A good doctor will always uphold principles of safety over and above everything else. A good doctor won't buy the cheapest Botox out there because he knows there may be a problem. The sad fact is, a lot of cosmetic devices and treatments don't work. A good doctor will be on the alert at all times and only use in the long run what he or she knows to be safe and effective."

Dr. Scott MacKenzie: Focus on the Patient

When I spoke to Scott MacKenzie by phone, I started by asking him, as I asked the other physicians I interviewed, why he thought people sought him out. Scott was unequivocal: it was word of mouth. Again and again my conversations with other cosmetic doctors have shown me that advertising is highly overrated. Rather, it's satisfied patients coming and going, patients who recognize that their doctor is concerned about them before anything else, that have built his reputation.

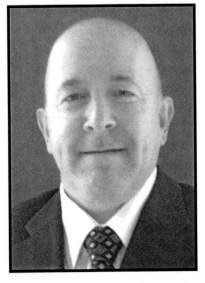

Scott MacKenzie is a highly respected cosmetic physician based in Corner Brook, Newfoundland, so far out in the Atlantic that it's closer to Europe than it is to most of the United States and Canada.

"The patient," he emphasized. "We must always be focused on the patient and what that patient would like done—*and* what's in their best interest. We must keep an open ear for their areas of concern. We have to listen at every stage to what the patient is looking for. We must maintain ethical standards of good care but, that said, we don't try to push our ideas or our thinking onto the patient."

Scott's talking about a technique that I refer to as reflective listening. It entails hearing the person but then offering a solution that's palatable to them, a solution that is the best of those available. But, as we've seen in other discussions, the options are constantly changing and the half-life of medical knowledge grows shorter and shorter.

Like some others I've spoken to, Scott is a member of my MasterMind group. He meets with my group of elite VIP doctors two or three times a year and these are all practicing cosmetic dermatologists, cosmetic surgeons and/or plastic surgeons.

...doctors in the cosmetic profession love to give back to society and love to share their abilities in other ways.

Remember the concept of sharing I mentioned? In this MasterMind group we share—something that doesn't always happen in medicine because doctors can be competitive and reluctant to tell all their secrets. When they get together, a unique feature of a MasterMind group is that the barriers come down and everybody starts chatting about everything.

Scott has found that too. "These groups are where you learn what's current, what's best, what's the latest. And when you really feel that you know those things, you have confidence as you deal with patients that you *can* provide the best."

It's just a fact of the real world that even when doctors are dealing with other, very good doctors in public forums such as conferences, what they hear from the podium may not be the whole truth. There are vested interests. That's why innovations such as the MasterMind groups appeal to the best doctors, who love the concept of sharing and are not easily made to feel insecure. MasterMind groups are the perfect setting for this.

It's been my experience that many of the doctors in the cosmetic profession love to give back to society and love to share their abilities in other ways. Scott MacKenzie is one of those who went to Africa and did surgery there for a period of time.

"I love to go to other parts of the world—most recently I was over in Kenya for a bit—where life may not be quite so rosy as it is for many of us here in North America. I love to go to these places and offer something of use to them. But you don't have to travel overseas. You can do it right here at home, as you do, Barry."

Scott and I talked about some of the characteristics of good cosmetic practitioners. We agreed that they tend to pay attention to the small things, the details and nuances in cosmetic procedures. This is important because, when we're doing a cosmetic procedure, it's the small things that matter. Many people can do the big things but it's actually the accumulation of little touches that can make a great result.

And as I noticed during other discussions, Scott emphasized that good communication with patients is a tremendous asset for anyone working in the cosmetic field.

"Just the process of simplification alone is critical," he said. "We never want to talk down to anybody but there's no need to use a lot of technical terminology. We're one person talking to another and in that respect we're on the same level.

"Sometimes patients come to me and they've already been seen by another cosmetic doctor. Quite often it's because they feel they weren't well-received or really respected or listened to. This is a communications issue."

The best way to listen is to be quiet for a while because most patients really need to be heard. When I asked Scott what factor might be most responsible for making his patients happy, he told me it was meeting their expectations, and he's been able to do that because he's heard their expectations and then delivered what they really wanted.

"And if we haven't been able to meet their expectations, I just honestly say, you know, we've tried our best. The important thing is that we didn't cut any corners. Complications can be a part of that picture."

Any surgeon who's been in practice for some time will have experienced some complications. The key to resolving these outcomes is the surgeon describing the procedure to the patient early on and in a fair bit of detail, including the things that may go wrong. This groundwork helps build trust before the procedure takes place and that trust can be very important in the unlikely event that a complication does occur. And if a complication does occur, a good doctor will be very direct, honest and forthright. That's what people are looking for more than anything. They don't want evasion.

All of us who have worked in clinics for a long time realize that it's not just the doctor but the other professionals that doctors surround themselves with who are important. Scott is a physician and surgeon and his wife is a registered nurse. She does many of the injectables and the Botox and various skin and laser procedures. After many years' experience and training, she's at a pretty high level. I call these people physician extenders because they do more than assist, they extend the physician's capacities to roles he or she could simply not accomplish alone.

"They've got that little bit more time than the doctor," Scott told me. "Time to maybe hang out with a patient and talk more with perhaps less pressure. Patients really appreciate that."

Like most physicians and surgeons, cosmetic practitioners like Scott are incredibly busy. But for many of them, their profession is also their passion. In fact, unless it's a passion, it's doubtful whether a cosmetic surgeon can do a great job. That's one difference between the best and the rest.

Daryl Hoffman: From Saving Limbs to Enhancing Lives

*D*r. Daryl Hoffman originally went to medical school to train as a psychiatrist but was seduced by what he learned about plastic surgery. He said "a lecturer in that subject, an alumnus of Stanford, so inspired him with his lectures about the fantastic possibilities of plastic surgery, I went to Stanford to study surgery, not psychiatry. I did a cosmetic fellowship in Miami and a fellowship on cleft lip in Tokyo. I then joined an organization that took me to various countries to perform charitable surgery for cleft lip and palate repair. In 1991 I joined a microsurgery practice here in Palo Alto and spent ten or fifteen years performing the kind of amazing procedures that had first inspired me in medical school. This work was largely non-elective—for the patient and me. 'This thoracic surgeon just took a six-inch chunk of skin, fat and rib out of this person,' they'd tell me. 'We want you to fix that.'

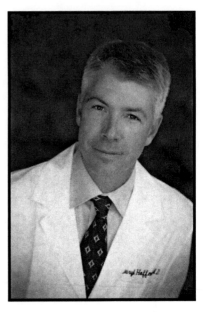

"As I got older, the long surgical hours—sometimes a procedure might require fifteen hours of standing—became more challenging. My microsurgery mentor, Dr. Kim, left to start a cosmetic practice. Over the next ten years or so, I myself evolved

Dr. Daryl Hoffman is a renowned cosmetic doctor based in Palo Alto, California, just outside San Francisco. He was originally from Los Alamos, New Mexico and began his medical training in his native state.

into a cosmetic surgeon. Maybe this evolution was made easier because the Silicon Valley is an affluent part of this country. But I feel that having that long background of salvaging disasters was what gave me the confidence to take a scalpel to a person who was perfectly well. I'd done it all before. I knew what was under there. An abdominoplasty was no great challenge.

"Today I'm really interested in the new and less invasive procedures that have emerged in recent years. These are the future of cosmetic surgery. If I was a patient, these are the procedures I'd want. As we get older, we yearn to slow the changes age brings but we're also averse to risk. Maybe we don't want our faces peeled back in order to look younger, especially not if there are alternatives. For a long time, non-invasive and minimally invasive treatments were not very effective. Now at last we seem to be on the verge of their becoming truly effective. Look at this new Cellulaze treatment for cellulite. It's not entirely non-invasive but it's a one-time treatment that's minimally invasive. Another example is breast augmentation by fat transfer. This is another minimally invasive procedure that's now been green-lighted by the American Society of Plastic Surgeons and may someday replace breast implants, which are potentially troublesome. These changes are pointing ahead."

"Today I'm really interested in the new and less invasive procedures that have emerged in recent years. These are the future of cosmetic surgery.

We turned to the challenge every patient faces: How do I find the best doctor for what I want? Daryl sympathizes with patients on this subject because he feels it's a difficult question for anyone to answer.

"To start with, what's right for one person may not be right for another. But one guideline is to consider the ultimate result. I personally don't like to look at somebody and say to myself, 'That person has had too much plastic surgery.' To be honest, people here in northern California laugh at the Los Angeles types with their cat-woman faces. I myself go to cosmetic surgery conventions and look at some of the wives and girl friends of surgeons and what do I see? I see people with too much access and not enough judgment. Their husbands didn't have enough judgment either, by the way—and that guy could be your cosmetic surgeon.

"So when you walk into a cosmetics office and the aesthetician and the consultant and the receptionist all have way too much Juvederm in their lips and their faces are a mask of cosmetic procedures that can hardly show expression, consider whether they share your values and aesthetics—or not. And by the way, almost everyone in the profession says they value naturalness, but in some

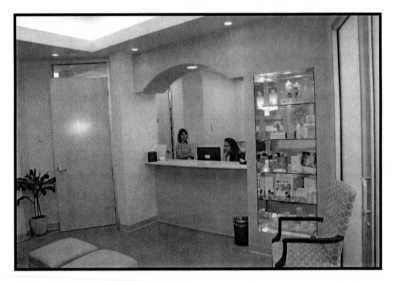

If it wasn't for the attractive case of cosmetic products, you might think Daryl Hoffman's reception area was that of any up-scale physician

cases you're entitled to wonder if they really do. These people seem to me to be influenced by the 'naturalness' professed by some of their patients—the 105-pound girl, for example, who really wants to be, like, natural but chooses double-D size implants. The moral: You want to come to a meeting of minds with the person you choose to perform your procedure. There are probably cosmetic surgeons who are not very good, but most—this is certainly true in this part of the country—most are well trained and good at what they do. So your challenge as a patient is usually to find a doctor you has the same aesthetic sense as you do. When you say, 'I want my face to look natural' and he agrees, you want to make sure you're talking about the same thing. I think my body of work is large enough and consistent enough that prospective patients can talk to other patients and look at photographs of my work and get an idea of my aesthetics. Sometimes there's a great meeting of minds and sometimes there's not. When there's not, I'd rather not do the operation. In fact, I've never been sorry for an operation I didn't do.

"As to finding that great fit, obviously a referral from a friend is no guarantee that his or her doctor is the doctor for you, but it certainly beats picking a billboard from the freeway. As a rule, a good place to *not* start is a chain that contracts its doctors or one that emphasizes the procedures rather than the people who do them. Yes, these are broad-brush guidelines and you might get lucky, but it's still a warning sign."

I and some other doctors have expressed our mistrust of doctor rating sites in no uncertain terms. But Daryl took a more nuanced stance.

"By all means, consult the popular ratings sites. Their shortcomings are obvious. One of my favourite Chinese restaurants just got slammed on Yelp. It's a great restaurant and the review just wasn't fair. No doctor wants to see that happen with his own reputation. But the fact is, these sites are here to stay and in the long run they make us all better. They keep everybody respectful of the fact that patients have a voice.

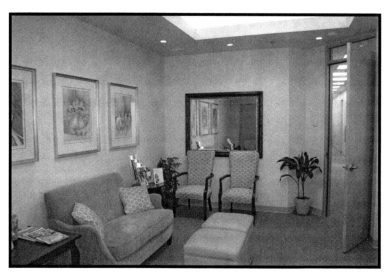

But when you turn the other way, the impression is more that of an executive suite. This attention to decorative detail is one of the tell-tale signs of good cosmetic surgeons

"As many doctors will tell you, you as a patient want someone with enough experience to be able to tell you what's going to
happen and with the ability to look after you if something does
go wrong. The old saw holds: 'Good judgment comes from experience and experience comes from bad judgment.'"

Ron Moy: Youthfulness from the Inside Out

*D*r. Ron Moy has been in cosmetic medicine for twenty-five
years, having begun his
training with two years as a
dermatology resident and two
years as a surgery resident focused on cosmetic and dermatological surgery. Today
he operates a clinic on Rodeo
Drive in Los Angeles.

"The field has changed so
rapidly that my early training is left far behind," he told
me. "We don't do anything
the way we did it twenty-five
or thirty years ago. I myself
have evolved into an anti-aging specialist and you can see
how that might be inevita-
ble for some of us. Our whole

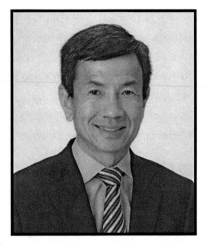

*Dr. Ron Moy is past president of the
American Academy of Dermatology
and a past president of the American
Society for Dermatologic Surgery.*

field is largely about slowing down the aging process. It goes
without saying that that's what external cosmetic procedures are
about, but I've found that we can achieve great results if we approach the challenge from the inside out. Think about how we
all look older when we're tired. In medical terms, correcting this
means addressing, say, possible sleep disorders. But we might
also be looking at adrenal fatigue or post-menopausal symptoms.

We might be looking at melatonin levels or other hormone levels. We might need to make use of DNA repair creams.

"None of this means I'm against performing lifts or resurfacings, but it does mean my group prefers to go for the underlying conditions first. This is not as common an approach as it might be because doctors are trained to treat disease, not retard aging."

At Ron Moy's practice, the clinicians approach anti-aging from an evidence-based perspective.

"Anti-oxidants, for instance. They're in almost every skin cream and on every supplement shelf in every drug store. But apart from the anti-oxidants in a good fruit and vegetable diet, no good study supports their use topically or as a supplement. That's why in our practice we use DNA-repair creams: their efficacy is supported by proper studies.

"After we've instituted a fairly complex anti-aging regimen for a patient, we may move on to the less invasive procedures: fat injections enriched with stem cells, resurfacing, filling, minimal tightening and neuromodulators like Botox. We believe that this approach, with its emphasis on a slowing of the aging process, in conjunction with the newer procedures, gives dramatically better results than the simple tightening of the skin."

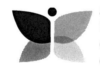

Anti-oxidants, for instance…are in almost every skin cream and on every supplement shelf.…But apart from the anti-oxidants in a good fruit and vegetable diet, no good study supports their use topically or as a supplement.

Signs Along the Way

I asked Ron what advice he'd give to someone who was in search of the ideal cosmetic practitioner. Not surprisingly, he favored practices that were in some way similar to his own broadly-based approach.

"Wherever you end up going, you want a wide variety of options. If you go to someone who just basically does Botox, you'll get what? Botox. What you want is a doctor—or group of doctors—who have lots of experience in lots of techniques. And remember that today we have a huge spectrum of effective equipment at our disposal. You don't want someone who has just one laser because lasers come in a huge variety to suit a range of applications. You want somebody who has a full armamentarium.

"The real point is this: a simple approach won't do because people—I mean our clients—don't fit easily into pigeon holes. This person might require volume added beneath the eyes, but the next person may require baggy tissue around the eyes to be removed.

"Obviously you want an experienced doctor with board certification, but beyond that, one of your first pointers should be referrals from friends who've already had an experience with a particular doctor. Then go and look at the practice's web site. A well-run web site may indicate a well-

Watch out, of course, for marketing that seems to over-promise.

run practice. Watch out, of course, for marketing that seems to over-promise. And check the doctor rating sites; they must be taken with a grain of salt but they're worth looking at. You might also check the regional medical board. I was on the California board for eight years and believe me, a medical board violation is to be taken seriously. Similarly, a lot of malpractice suits are hardly a good sign."

Every colleague I spoke to put emphasis on the personal consultation as a valuable tool for prospective patients, especially in the case of more complex procedures. Ron Moy especially emphasizes the significance of attractive premises, offices and surgical facilities, and he reminds us that the staff is responsible for much of the care you'll receive. A courteous staff is a key to a good experience. "And," he added, "the doctor too. His or her manner and approach is at the center of the whole thing."

As my readers know, I'm a believer in doctors' community work as an indicator of their attitudes towards patients. Ron Moy is himself a community volunteer and has worked as a doctor in Peru in a volunteer capacity. But he pointed out that there are good doctors who are not volunteers. No rule can be 100% reliable. I myself have never put much stress on a doctor's leadership in professional organizations, but Ron, who has a distinguished history of organizational work, reminded me that you don't get to head a professional group without being ethical and empathetic. It is, as he said, a kind of peer review.

"And this is important, because there are doctors in this field who perform unnecessary procedures. That's one of the reasons medicine in the U.S. is so expensive."

Steven Schlosser: Trust

Steve studied medicine at Georgetown and trained at Tufts. Now sixty-four, he practiced obstetrics and general and gynecological surgery (OBGYN) in Los Angeles for almost twenty-five years and delivered some 3000 babies. Then, in the early 2000s, he changed his career direction.

"We had our son quite late—I was forty-seven. I'd waited a long time for him and I didn't want to miss his childhood. I decided I wanted to do something that wouldn't involve getting called out at nights. About this time

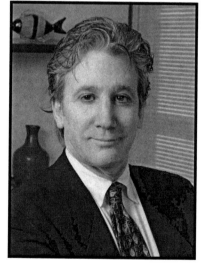

Respected cosmetic surgeon Dr. Steven Schlosser has devoted serious attention to the dilemma patients face when searching for the qualified practitioner who best suits their needs.

cosmetics were just becoming a huge topic and it seemed to me a natural fit and something I'd enjoy doing. That proved to be the case.

Actually, as Steve explained, the transition from OBGYN to cosmetics is fairly common.

"People in the OBGYN field are very comfortable talking to women and dealing with their medical problems—and women still constitute the majority of cosmetic patients.

"The fact is, cosmetic surgeons are generally tremendously enthusiastic about their work. Not only is it gratifying to be reliably paid for hard work—and that's often not the case in the U.S. medical system—but the enormous variety of new techniques—the injectable procedures, the skin procedures, the body sculpture—is really stimulating. Some doctors go all the way to breast surgery and face lifts but all these techniques have to be learned along the way. Even the reconstructive training that plastic surgeons receive does not fully prepare them for cosmetic work. New procedures seem to emerge every six months. We're all talking about the 'Cellulaze' treatment for cellulite, for example. It's brand new and looks like it's going to be a home run.

"When I made the late decision to enter cosmetics, I moved to Boulder, Colorado and opened a 3500-square-foot clinic with five staff to help me. We've been successful and received a number of awards."

Due Diligence in Three Stages

I turned to the challenge patients face when deciding on a cosmetic doctor. Steve divides the process into three stages.

"Every stage is a form of due diligence and your goal is to avoid two common mistakes. The first mistake is falling into the hands of an inexperienced practitioner. The encounter might be good for him—he's learning, after all—but not so good for you the patient. The second mistake is to confuse cosmetic surgery with a Costco product. Your goal should not be to find the cheapest.

Cheapness is in fact a worrying sign that could mean several things, including inexperience on the doctor's part, the very thing you are trying to avoid.

"The first stage of your due diligence, as you begin to explore your options, begins ideally by talking to friends and colleagues who've had cosmetic work done of the type you want. The limitation is that many people are reluctant to discuss their experiences. I have many patients who've been delighted with their outcomes but who'll never tell anyone about it.

"Even if no one you know is prepared to share information, you'll find television shows and whole magazines devoted to the subject, and some of these are truly cutting edge. But if you find you have a serious interest in this subject, the Internet is your best friend.

"You have a problem; let's say it's brown spots. You type "brown spots" into a search and immediately a whole world opens up: procedures, doctors, technical companies. It's overwhelming but you can quickly refine the results. It's probably not the technical equipment makers that you're interested in. The various brown-spot procedures are important, of course, and reading about them gives you something of a handle on the subject. Then there are the doctors who treat brown spots: you're inter- …many other procedures call for no specific background but, of course, are better always performed by experienced practitioners.

ested in those in your area, not the ones in Brazil. And you'll want to go further. I've found that many patients are prepared to conduct quite sophisticated due diligence. They'll look into a doctor's background. Is he a dermatologist? A family doctor? An OBGYN? A general surgeon? This can matter because some procedures require special skills, others not. Only a plastic surgeon is likely to be trained properly to do a nose job. Only a dermatologist is likely to do Mohs surgery for skin cancer. And many other procedures call for no specific background but, of course, are better always performed by experienced practitioners.

"You can search the doctor's name and explore the on-line rating sites to see what people are saying about this doctor. There are a lot of these sites; you can find them at google.com, at realself. com, at locateadoc.com and elsewhere. Check them out without lending too much weight to any one. If you go to a bunch of sites and they all rate a specific doctor highly, that's a good sign. A lot of bad opinion naturally raises a question. I've found that most patients who come to me have already checked those sites and have been reassured by what they've read. It's true that an angry patient can publically besmirch a doctor and of course that makes doctors nervous. But an angry or unhappy patient should be a matter of concern. Doctors are perfectly able to contact such a patient and do whatever's possible to correct the problem.

"Okay, so you've searched around and checked out reputations. Now go to the doctor's own web site. These sites can tell you a lot. Is it warm, informative, comprehensive, easy to use? An excellent site suggests a professional practice. A meager little site suggests a modest practice that may not be able to meet your needs.

"Now you've gathered information about relevant procedures and several doctors, you can pick, say, three and begin to compare them. First, call the offices to schedule a consultation. Use this call to ask some questions of whomever you're speaking to. Some practices will tell you a lot over the phone, others not. Whatever the case, ask them to send you their information package by mail. These packages should provide you with a detailed menu of their services, perhaps some articles by the doctor, perhaps photos or even a book if the doctor has written one. Reading this material and comparing completes your first stage.

Steve's second stage of due diligence is of course the actual visit to the doctor's office.

"Look around critically. Is the overall impression more spa-like than medical? The question might seem like a strange one—after all, you are seeing a doctor—but the fact is that when doctors fully commit to a cosmetic practice, they tend to upgrade their offices to reflect this emphasis on aesthetics. A "medical"-looking office may suggest that a doctor is still new to cosmetics or not yet fully committed.

"Observe the staff. Are they friendly? Are they warm, kind, knowledgeable, informative and attentive? Or are they just rushing around engaged in their tasks? The staff is going to be a big part of your experience if you do choose this clinic."

But should a prospective patient expect to see the doctor on this visit?

"It depends. If you're there for skin services, meeting the doc-

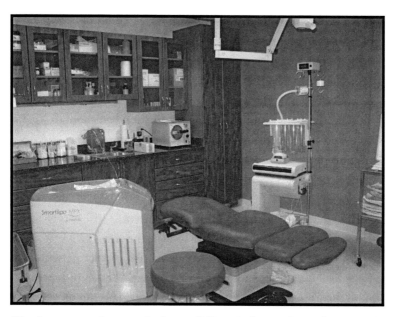

The elegant operating room in Steven Schlosser's Avanti clinic tells you much about the sort of quality facility you're visiting.

tor may not be necessary. But if you're there for surgery, it is necessary. Whatever the case, remember to ask how many cases the doctor has handled. Has he or she done it seven times? Fifty times? A thousand times? Bear in mind that many procedures are quite new: Smart Lipo, for example, is only four or five years old. When did this doctor start doing it? And, by the way, is he or she board certified? When did he or she receive that certification? This information has to be put in context, of course. A doctor doesn't have to be a certified plastic surgeon to do body sculpting because a plastic surgeon's training doesn't include that sort of training anyway.

"If you haven't received all the available brochures and materials before this consultation visit, now is the time to get them. The same is true of patient testimonials,

...ask how many cases the doctor has handled. Has he or she done it seven times? Fifty times? A thousand times?

which are critically important to your decision. If you haven't seen them already, they should be available at the office in a book or collection of some sort.

"And the only thing more important than testimonials are before-and-after pictures. You should be able to see big, high-resolution photos of work performed by this doctor and in the area you're concerned with. And make sure they are his pictures, not someone else's."

But what if after all this effort, the patient is still sitting on the fence, unable to decide whether to take the plunge?

"In that case, ask to speak to one or two former patients who have had your procedure performed. Most offices will accommodate this. It's the ultimate "eye-witness" evidence."

"But in the end, all your information and questions, with the responses you've received, add up to one thing: your trust. Would you trust this doctor to look after you? Do you believe he or she cares? If the answer is yes, you've found your doctor."

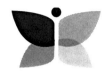

3 WHAT PATIENTS SAY

fter speaking with my distinguished colleagues—those we've just met and others I wasn't able to include—I realized there was an important perspective missing. No matter how hard I and other surgeons try, we tend to see our profession from our own perspective. I may not know exactly what answers I'm going to get from Ron Moy or Jeff Riopelle, but I can make a pretty good guess: the same experiences and influences that have shaped my attitudes have shaped theirs.

So I turned to our patients, people for whom (with one notable exception) cosmetic surgery is not part of daily life but a unique and potentially daunting experience. These are the people I saw a few times in my office and again for follow-ups and then perhaps not again for a very long time. What did it all mean to them and what could they say to others who were considering taking the same step?

I canvassed my own patients, of course. Anything else would be unethical. Some of them, in talking about their experiences, say some things that are slightly embarrassing to me—though not in a bad way. But that's part of their story and I've let them do the talking. I've changed only their names.

Rachel, 72

I'm a fit and active woman who runs and works out regularly. People are always saying, "Oh, you look so good!" and I'm thinking, "Maybe my body is firm but there are no elliptical machines for the face."

Let's be honest: I'm a woman and I'm seventy-two years old and I'm as vain as many of us. As we get older, we get wrinkles and deep creases and start to look all puckered. I just didn't want that.

I'd had a little exposure to cosmetic procedures. I'd had my eyes done successfully about fifteen years earlier and I'd tried Botox about six years ago. I had a vague awareness of these new fillers. But it was when I received a flyer announcing one of Barry Lycka's seminars and went along, perhaps more because I was interested in the spa that was sharing the event with him, that the light went on for me. The presentation impressed me and I decided to take up the offer of a free consultation.

I'm a woman and I'm seventy-two years old and I'm as vain as many of us. As we get older, we get wrinkles and deep creases and start to look all puckered. I just didn't want that.

My cosmetic surgeon himself is a lovely man. We discussed the various options and I decided to go for the Sculptra "plump-up" filler and scheduled the first session for about a month later. I was a bit apprehensive, of course, because it was new to me and I realized it would involve inserting needles around sensitive areas like the eyes and mouth, but a local anesthetic numbed my face and the nurse was very reassuring. even if I squeezed her hand so hard she must have worried I'd take her fingers with me.

My doctor took only about five minutes to do the actual injections. The level of discomfort I'd compare to a ' flu shot. I went back once a month for the next five months. In the interval between the shots the Sculptra gradually spreads and lifts the muscles and skin to diminish and even eradicate creases and wrinkles. The result is at least as good as Botox without Botox's drawbacks and is expected to last several years with maybe some annual tweaks.

The result? I look in the mirror and kiss myself every morning. The look is subtle, natural and exactly what I wanted.

Did I recommend it to anyone else? And put up with people criticizing and commenting? No. It's nobody's business. Okay, I told one friend and she then went in for a partial treatment and she was happy too.

Mary, 51

I'm a fifty-one-year-old entrepreneur and I've just incorporated a new software company this year. My role is that of sole interface with our customers. One day not long ago I was talking to a client and mentioned that I was going to get my hair done.

"They always want to see a young 'you,' don't they?" he said.

I thought, "He's right. But how far do you go?"

I'd had no previous exposure to anything like cosmetic surgery except for a breast reduction years ago, which was done for medical reasons. As I approached fifty, I realized I was concerned about my thighs: it was a very private concern because no one knew or cared. If I did anything about the problem, it would just be for me—and maybe my husband, who's never said anything negative.

I'd heard ads for my cosmetic surgeon's clinic on the radio for a couple of years but I was reluctant to make the leap. Finally in the summer of 2011, I went along for a consultation. Nine days later, after a ton of paperwork, I had the procedure.

My doctor's appearance and demeanor are perfect for his role. When you meet him, your first reaction is to feel comfortable. You're vulnerable in a situation like this and the last thing you need is somebody who looks—or wants to look—like Adonis. You just wouldn't go through with it. Barry's personal presentation is modest and he clearly picked his young staff with great care. They're totally welcoming and accepting. My only concern was that the receptionist booking the procedure had to do so within earshot of others sitting in the reception area. I know my doctor would care about that sort of thing, which is why I mention it.

I can't describe the liposuction procedure as painless. I experienced major discomfort but was able to breathe my way through it and stay perfectly still the whole time. That's important for the surgeon. But to keep this in perspective, I should add that I could have driven home afterwards if I'd needed to, and the very next day I accompanied my mom on a shopping trip to Costco. As to downtime—there was none, really. I wore a Spanks garment—a sort of girdle—under my clothes for a few days after.

But after four weeks, when I went back for a reassessment, he took pictures and we compared them with the pictures taken before the procedure. The difference was astonishing.

The effects appeared gradually as the swelling went down. You see yourself every day, of course, and I didn't see anything dramatic. But after four weeks, when I went back for a reassessment, he took pictures and we compared them with the pictures taken before the procedure. The difference was astonishing. In fact, I understand that it can take up to a year for the whole transformation to take place. The body is still absorbing fat and the skin, which is still elastic, gradually sucks back in.

How do I feel about in now, months later? I'm thrilled. This was something I did for myself, as I said, not for others. Certainly it was great to see the difference in the pictures, but for me the important things were more subtle. When I put on my skinny jeans, there's a gap between my thighs that wasn't there before. And I'm not going to go into detail about this, but both my husband and I noticed a subtle improvement in our love making. These changes are nonetheless enormously important for me.

That's what's significant about my doctor's approach and that of his staff. The emphasis is not on being perfect but on being the best you—whatever that means to you. My only regret is that this kind of procedure isn't affordable for more people. I'm afraid that accounts for some of the negative publicity that gets pointed at cosmetic procedures.

If you're thinking about having a procedure done, it's incredibly important to do your homework. I'm not saying this because of things I've read: it's based on my experience with my own family. Both my sisters, who are about my age, are spending immense sums on resurfacing procedures—laser in one case, peels in the other. In both cases, they're going to little tiny places here in town and I'm seriously dubious about the value they're getting for their money. Why wouldn't I refer them to my doctor, you ask? One of my sisters did see Barry about wrinkles above her lip. Here's the key point: my doctor wouldn't do it unless she had more extensive treatment because, as he told her, it would make her look funny. She couldn't afford more than just the immediate lip area so that was that. Really, that's what's so cool about his approach. My doctor refused to do what she wanted because he knew it wasn't the right course.

Christine, 43

*Y*ou have to remember when you're talking about cosmetic procedures that sometimes there's more at stake than looks. You have to remember that many practitioners such as my doctor are medical professionals, not just people who can improve your appearance.

In 2003 I began to notice a small, orange-colored spot on one cheek. It was sort of itchy and it didn't go away. A similar rough, thick patch appeared on the other cheek. I started to find this embarrassing because it was pretty much impossible to cover these spots with make-up. Doctors started commenting and even my dentist mentioned the first spot, though nobody knew what it was. Finally, in 2007, I visited my doctor's office to see if he could remove it. He examined it really carefully.

"Hmmmm," he said. "I'm quite sure this is an amyloid."

Of course I'd never heard of such a thing; it is so rare, most doctors have never seen an amyloid.

"I'm going to send you to a specialist at University Hospital," My doctor said.

Amyloidosis can be a terrible disease if it affects an internal organ. Once it appears on, say, the liver or the heart, it can grow rapidly and destroy the organ before anything can be done. In this way, it's something like cancer.

At University Hospital, Edmonton, a biopsy confirmed amyloidosis but their tests didn't turn up any signs of the disease in my blood or bone marrow. From then on, they regularly monitored me but the diagnosis was localized amyloidosis.

By 2011, I was back where I'd started eight years earlier: alive and well but with these unsightly lesions growing larger on my face. I went back to my doctor. He was very cautious and did his own research. Finally he said, "I can try but no guarantees. I'm just going to do a test."

He got on the Internet at 3 A.M. one morning and consulted on my behalf with a doctor in

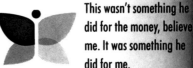

This wasn't something he did for the money, believe me. It was something he did for me.

Pennsylvania, a world expert in amyloid. Then, in August of 2011, he treated one spot with a UPL laser. Of course these lasers weren't designed for this purpose but my doctor decided it might just be effective. Two weeks later, when the redness from the treatment began to fade, we could already see the heavy, thick amyloid tissue was gone. He then did the other cheek.

Since then, my doctor has monitored the result of his "test." This wasn't something he did for the money, believe me. It was something he did for me. And as you can see, this story also shows that he wasn't concerned only with appearance but with my real health and safety.

Jessica, 46

I'm forty-six now and live in a major city. I grew up in a small tourist town and was Mrs. Canada International in 2003. My mom and my aunt both had face lifts that changed their lives and I myself had a rhinoplasty procedure when I was nineteen. It was successful but the surgeon didn't attempt to correct a deviated septum I was born with. I remained a mouth breather all my life until years later, a well-known plastic surgeon, corrected the septum so I could breathe properly and made some cosmetic improvements to the nose.

More recently, I'd been troubled by frown lines between my eyes. My plastic surgeon referred me to another doctor, whom she knew. This doctor treated the frown lines with Botox but unfortunately my high metabolism pretty much works Botox out of my system right away. I attended another doctor's information sessions. About one hundred people showed up and each one paid $25, which this doctor donates to a cancer charity. When the session was over, I spoke to him and told him about the problem. He said, "There's a new product on the market. come and see me and we'll talk."

I went along and he explained that this product, Xeomin, which is claimed as an improvement on Botox, was new to him and if I would like to try it, he'd do it for free.

My other areas of concern were "Pinocchio" lines around my mouth, and lines above the upper lip that draw lipstick, and a slightly sunken area under both eyes. This doctor proposed to use a filler called Restylane on all these areas and the new Xeomin between the eyes.

For most people, Xeomin is supposed to work for three to six months, but on me it faded fairly quickly, as Botox had. That's why the offer to try it for free was so welcome. The filler on the other hand worked really well. My doctor did something of a touch-up afterwards. Restylane is expensive and he never described it as permanent. It's fading a bit now, some months later, but I'm very pleased: there's no lipstick bleed and I've got my 25-year-old eyes back. Nobody says, "Jessica, you look so tired," anymore.

I know cosmetic procedures are sniffed at in some circles. In some ways, it's like attitudes towards fur coats. I'm a tall woman who wears fur. When I'm walking down the main street in my town, I get various looks from various age groups. That's why you need to wear fur with confidence and it's ditto for cosmetic procedures. I'm a successful salesperson and I need to feel confident about what I see when I look at myself. Other people's reactions to my cosmetic work—if they happen to know about it—range from eager curiosity to faint scorn. But for me, those are like reactions to my fur coat—or my ten-year-old car: I don't care one way or the other. Some people choose to make over their kitchen. I choose to look younger. Subtlety and naturalness is what modern cosmetic work is all about. My doctor's emphasis is all that way. Actresses who go around with their lips pumped up are making a mockery of their beauty.

Of course the simple fact—never mind vanity—is that our sales clients prefer to deal with good-looking people, so improving my appearance is a work bonus. Sales is a man's world and if necessary I'll use my looks and sexuality to make a sale.

Sadly, some of these procedures can be cost-prohibitive. There are so many women out there who'd do what I did if they could afford it, although maybe they wouldn't tell anybody.

Deirdre, 44

I'm a forty-four-year-old woman, fit and petite at 4'11" and 100 pounds—my weight since I was eighteen. I've always been very physical, the kind of person, who, if you needed a piano moved, I'd move it.

Several years ago, when I was getting maybe five hours of exercise a day, my upper body was rock solid. Unfortunately, I'd inherited plump thighs from my Ukrainian grandma. I want to make it clear: no one was complaining about my thighs; they were something that bothered me and me only because they just didn't seem to fit with the rest of my body.

I really knew nothing about cosmetic procedures. A few people in my acquaintance had had breast augmentation surgery but that was far from anything that would interest me. But some time about 2008, I saw a program on the new laser liposuction and learned that a local cosmetic doctor was among the pioneers using this technology in the world.

Once I had this information, I didn't hesitate. This doctor is a familiar name here and I trusted the man even before I met him. I was confident that it would go well for me. My attitude frankly was "How could the removal of excess fat be a bad thing?"

I should remind you that liposuction is not designed as a weight-loss program. I wouldn't want my before-and-after photos to give lazy people the wrong idea. I'd done everything possible with those thighs.

During my first consultation, the doctor's staff discussed the options I had: basically conventional liposuction or the new laser liposuction. The conventional procedure would have required me to go back several times over a period of six months or a year. It's a more invasive procedure that costs somewhat less and if it had been the only option, I probably would have decided against it. It was the laser option I wanted and when my doctor examined my thighs, he said this technology was made for people like me.

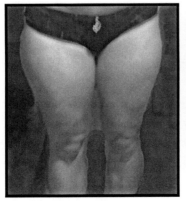 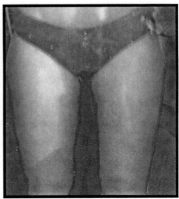

Deirdre before   *Deirdre after*

"This procedure changed my level of self-esteem so dramatically, it didn't matter that nobody else had been concerned about my thighs. I had done it for myself." —Deirdre

The operation was booked for about four months from my consultation but just two weeks later, when I still hadn't fully committed to going ahead, his office called me and said they'd had a cancellation for the following Monday. There was no putting it off. "Yes," I said.

The procedure is performed under a local anesthetic but there is still pain associated with it.

I should remind you that liposuction is not designed as a weight-loss program....I'd done everything possible with those thighs.

Liposuction is not something for people with no tolerance whatsoever for pain. It is however the sort of pain you can bear down and deal with because you know benefits are going to flow from it. When it was over, my doctor expressed some surprise at the amount of fat the process had removed; I seem to recall it was something like two litres. I'd taken a photograph of myself in my bedroom the morning of the procedure. Although it was important to keep the pressure dressings on for a few days, I did take them off briefly the first night after the procedure. That's when I took the second, dramatically different photo. In some cases, the results can improve over a period of months, but in my case, the optimal result was reached within a week or two.

This procedure changed my level of self-esteem so dramatically, it didn't matter that nobody else had been concerned about my thighs. I had done it for myself.

Seymour, 65

I'm a sixty-five-year-old psychologist with thirty years experience in the clinical and consulting field. Some years ago I noticed I'd become increasingly bothered by the way my face had changed with age to produce puffy bulges in my lower cheeks, one on each side. I have quite high cheekbones but beneath there was something of a hollow and then these chipmunk pouches, as I called them.

My doctor is among the top two or three cosmetic practitioners in my city and his media profile is fairly high, with radio and TV appearances and information sessions on a regular basis. I didn't actually know anyone—no man anyway—who had had a cosmetic procedure, but maybe the fact that the clinic was on the same floor as my office was a factor. I went in for a consultation based on this and on his excellent reputation. He provided me with a range of options and described the effect and duration of each. Sculptra seemed to offer a longer effect—as much as two years—with the added advantage of stimulating natural collagen development.

I had two sessions, perhaps six weeks apart. My doctor used Sculptra to fill in around my eyes and mouth to achieve a smoothing out of my face. After the second session, I couldn't see anything more that needed to be done. The effect was remarkable and as a side benefit, I looked ten to fifteen years younger. I was delighted and there's no doubt that the procedure has had a beneficial effect on my clinical practice.

There doesn't seem to be any competition between my doctor and the other top practitioners. He simply invests in the best equipment and strives to provide superb service as his duty to his patients. His staff—both nursing and non-nursing—is exceptionally helpful and congenial. It was as though his people liked to pamper. What might have been a potentially discomforting procedure became a somewhat enjoyable experience. As each needle went in, I said to myself, "This is going to make a big difference."

The doctor can only inject in so many sites—you can't have a hundred needles stuck in your face—so afterwards there's a gradual improvement over time as the filler evens out. The results have remained stable for almost two years and only recently have I noticed that it was time for a touch-up.

This sort of injected filler treatment is cost-effective and less likely to cause anxiety than more radical procedures. A few injections can bring a great deal of satisfaction. People these days are generally more inclined to little-at-a-time procedures rather than dramatic and sudden change, with its attendant risks.

I didn't disclose to others the fact that I'd had this work done, but I have sometimes recommended my doctor to patients who expressed any preoccupation with aging. Some of these people have followed my suggestion and reported happy results. A minority are men but why shouldn't men reap these benefits? Men have many of the same motivations women have. I hope to inspire others to forego their hesitations and reservations and explore the possibilities of appropriate cosmetic procedures. People like my doctor have the sort of magic touch that can make almost anyone beautiful—or more beautiful.

The Experience

I can almost hear you thinking: "Right. Those are the successful ones. What about the others?"

Part of my professional work is not to undertake procedures that are inappropriate or that will tend to result in likely disappointment. I don't have to do any procedure against my will and I won't. I try to think of my patients as members of my family: If my aunt asked me to do this and I thought she wouldn't be happy—or I wouldn't be—I wouldn't do it for her. And I wouldn't do it for you either.

Rather unexpectedly, my interest in patients' stories led me to one of the ultimate cosmetic surgery stories, one more interesting and complex than its frequent media airings would suggest. It's a story that reminds us all of the critical meeting place between cosmetic surgery and important medical intervention, reminds us that when we say we're going to "let nature take its course" we may not be thinking it through all the way. It's also a testimony to resilience in the face of setbacks few of us have had to face and overcome.

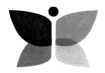

4 SARAH BURGE
THE PATIENT AS CONSULTANT

ike most of medicine, cosmetic surgery addresses a wide spectrum, from crises tied to the very physical and mental well-being of patients to complaints that are more a matter of whim and require interventions that are perhaps ill-advised. As a long-practicing surgeon, I'm accustomed to threading my way through my patients' hopes, needs and wishes, trying to make the recommendations I believe will serve them best.

The challenge is all the greater because cosmetic medicine consists of so many different techniques, some requiring much skill and experience, others more easily mastered. A patient may be quite unsuitable for one procedure but a perfect candidate for another. A practitioner may be a master of one but largely unfamiliar with another.

I don't normally give these matters much thought. From day to day, my professional career tends to be filled with the joy of helping people whose lives are marred by unhappiness that stems from a cosmetic problem. Whether I'm subtly re-contouring a healthy patient's face or tummy to restore her or his pride in her or his physical appearance, or removing the stigma of a tattoo from a former prostitute or rebuilding the face of a battered woman, my work is about human happiness, not extreme vanity or psychological obsession. But it was a particular case—my reconstruction of

Elizabeth Russell's broken features, the result of a terrible beating by an abusive partner—that reawakened these issues.

In about 2000 or 2001, I had heard about Elizabeth, a courageous woman whose dreadfully damaged features had taken her out of the mainstream of life. I decided to offer her a series of pro bono surgical procedures through which she might reclaim that life. Great North Productions, with the support of the Canadian government, documented the story, which was shown on the Life Network and eventually released on YouTube. By 2001, Elizabeth had been liberated from the scars of her past and had proudly returned to the workplace. Recently, a colleague who knew this story contacted me.

"Have you heard about Sarah Burge?" he asked.

The name sounded vaguely familiar.

"Who?"

"Sarah Burge. The Real-Life Barbie."

"Oh oh. Maybe."

"She's got a book out— *The Half a Million Pound Girl.*"

"Let me guess."

"Exactly. It's the value of her cosmetic surgery."

This woman, whose seemingly glitzy story and scandalous forthrightness in advocating for cosmetic surgery, was to re-awaken my interest in the public's perception of my profession.

Now I remembered the stories. The woman who'd had more cosmetic surgery than anyone on the planet. And some scandal too. Something about her giving her nine-year-old daughter a gift certificate for cosmetic surgery and teaching her to pole dance.

"What's going to surprise you, Barry, is that Sarah Burge is another Elizabeth Russell case."

This conversation was the link that began my interest in a person I might never have dreamed of speaking to, never mind coming to know. This woman, whose seemingly glitzy story and scandalous forthrightness in advocating for cosmetic surgery, was to re-awaken my interest in the public's perception of my pro-fession—and in my profession's perception of itself. As I was to learn, her extraordinary verve had taken her beyond recovery to add a new dimension to cosmetic medicine: the cosmetic surgery consultant.

Sarah Burge is a celebrity of sorts. At the very least she's known all over the world to anyone interested in cosmetic surgery. Feed-ing this celebrity are a series of stories about her past, her amazing appetite for cosmetic procedures, and her reputed advocacy of cos-metic procedures for minors. So what was behind all this?

By the time I interviewed Sarah at her home in England, I'd started to read her book and saw that my colleague was right: she'd indeed been a victim. Like many women who'd suffered her fate, she had combined a secret fascination with "bad" men and a curious naiveté. Her part-time fling, so charming, turned sud-denly on her for the overt sexiness that was part of her persona. When she protested, he attacked her with brutal misogynist fe-rocity, breaking her teeth, the bones of her face and hands in what appears to have been a murder attempt, then walked away, leav-ing her lying shattered in the street. She spent weeks in hospital as doctors and surgeons worked to save her life and patch her body and face together.

During the year that followed, as she painfully recovered, she received a diagnosis of multiple sclerosis, and at the end of that year, incredibly but not unprecedentedly in such situations, she re-turned to the man who had so abused her. She was to remain with him for another ten years, still subjected to his beatings.

This sad story might have ended here, very much where Eliza-beth was when I intervened to repair her looks after similar abuse. But my interest in Sarah's story was on another account altogeth-er. I had learned that, at this point in her life, she had made deci-sions that would lead her into the world of cosmetic surgery and not ultimately as a patient but as a contributor.

Sarah began in 1990 to train as a beautician, taking one course after another in advanced and semi-permanent make-up. She boldly approached Britain's cosmetic surgery elite on Harley Street, offering to assist with post-operative make-up and care. She had no takers, but undeterred she eventually rented space on Harley Street itself, opening a practice by offering various resurfacing and minor cosmetic procedures as she gained the necessary qualifications. Meanwhile, she familiarized herself with the doctors around her, determining who was best at what. From these beginnings, she made the next leap. She opened a salon in the suburb of Pinner and was soon knocking on the doors of Harley Street again. This time her strategy was to effectively offer herself as a "human guinea pig." If surgeons would work to improve her battered appearance, she would refer potential patients to them. Since at that time British doctors were forbidden by law to advertise, such informed referrals were of considerable value. At first she was rewarded with modest discounts on her own cosmetic work, but the relationships became more business-like with time—and Sarah Burge's face was eventually restored to her satisfaction.

The turmoil of her personal life was finally resolved when she married her childhood sweetheart, Tony Burge. But no sooner had she embarked on this new and quieter life than she was charged with benefit fraud. The case ended with the judge requiring her to repay the sum in question, but the resilient Sarah, at first crushed and defeated, managed once again to transform her circumstances. The case had centered around the accusation that she had used benefits money to pay for her extensive surgery. She was forced to close her salon and found herself hounded by the media, who seemed interested only in her cosmetic surgery history. It was *The Mirror*—a London tabloid—that ran the story branding her "the £100,000 Real-Life Barbie." ("Actually," Sarah told me, "as a kid I never liked Barbie.")

From these beginnings flowed a world-wide stream of publicity—and ironically it was on the basis of this publicity that Sarah

Burge has made her contribution to cosmetic medicine.

The subject of this book is your choice of a cosmetic surgeon. We've seen how surgeons themselves are conscious of the difficulty of that choice. A person seeking a cosmetic procedure can hardly expect a surgeon to answer the question, "Are you the best?" (That's why, at the end of the book, I've included The Doctor Index to help provide the answer.) We've also seen how first-hand experience and personal referrals are a useful guide. If you have a friend who's undergone a successful liposuction, you'll take her referral seriously. But what are your choices if you have no such friends? This is where encountering Sarah Burge and learning about her history provided real insight.

As Sarah acquired ever greater experience with cosmetic medicine, both as a patient and as a Harley Street neighbor to some of that country's best surgeons, she saw a need.

"Look," she said. "I get thousands of e-mails every year from distressed persons seeking a solution to cosmetic problems that make them truly unhappy. Some of these people are desperate. As the years have gone by, I've learned more and more how to help them."

She was sitting on the opposite side of a table in a pub near her home not far from Cambridge, England. Beside her was her husband Tony. She looked a comfortable decade or two younger than her fifty-year-old self.

"First, there is the question of competency on the part of the professionals performing the procedures. I'm not just talking about the voodoo-witch-doctor types lurking in various corners—people who may have no proper medical training at all and are actually engaged in a sort of medical fraud. They exist, though thankfully not in great numbers. I'm also talking about young and inexperienced surgeons just out of school. They need to learn—fair enough—but they must learn under careful supervision and you as the patient need to know if they're learning on *you*.

"The problem is that these legitimate but less experienced

practitioners work for less money and are commonly recruited by big cosmetic surgery firms that work strictly for the bottom line. These firms may be just the ones that can afford the more aggressive advertising and are likely to attract the largest number of clients. How is a person to know?

"And it's worrying, but inexperience isn't the only problem among officially qualified doctors. The plain fact is that this is a constantly evolving field and surgeons must be constantly refreshing their knowledge and taking courses in new technologies and procedures. And some surgeons—stick-in-the-muds young and old—just don't. How is a patient to know that? Because even if you ask, how can you judge the answers?"

As the stream of publicity continued and her reputation—notoriety in the eyes of some—grew, and more people sought her opinion, Sarah took the same approach to assessing practitioners that any prudent patient might if The plain fact is that this is a constantly evolving field and surgeons must be constantly refreshing their knowledge and taking courses in new technologies and procedures.

they only could: she observed procedures and follow-ups. She observed the preparations and the outcomes. She took note of who was good and at what—after all, who better than a patient to assess an outcome?—and which surgeon would best fit a particular need. And now, as she continued to counsel prospective patients, she found herself drawn into a more involved role.

"People needed help. They needed that first stage of advice: 'This will probably respond to laser therapy' or 'This will probably require a filler' or 'It's a facelift you're looking for.' But when I'd place a client with a surgeon, I found that in many cases, post-operatively, the surgeon was relying on his receptionist to deal with patient queries. Patients had no hope of ever getting the man himself back on the phone. I needed to be there to counsel and support.

"This was all the more important when I'd hear from people who'd gone off to some far-away place for a bargain procedure. Even now we see people flying straight back from tummy tuck operations in eastern Europe—people who should be in bed.

"All this points to the need for considerable follow-up support for some cosmetic procedures—not in every case but in a significant number. The best clinics and surgeons provide this support but others don't—and that's where I come in.

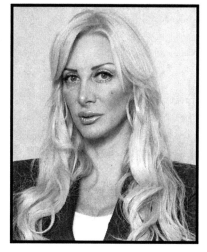

"I'm sorry to say this, but the role of independent cosmetic surgery consultant—a role I'm partly responsible for creating—is so much in demand that unqualified persons are stepping in there too. Some firms are paying hairdressers and such for referrals. This is just business—I understand that—but it offers no solution."

The more I talked to Sarah Burge, the more I appreciated that she was no safety scold trying to frighten people into engaging her services.

Sarah Burge. Once a victim, then a cosmetic patient, then a cosmetic surgery advocate, now a cosmetic surgery consultant.

"People approach this field with huge fear," she said. "Fear of a catastrophe on the operating table, fear of pain, fear of permanent damage. These fears are largely unfounded. The risks associated with professional, experienced procedures are very low. It's sometimes necessary to adjust a result in some way but that's part of the process and every good surgeon is equipped to do that. I do advise all my clients to refrain from general anesthetic. Modern cosmetic procedures rarely require it and it poses dangers that have nothing to do with cosmetic surgery itself—but apart from that, once you've found the right doctor, you can expect a good outcome."

My conversations with Sarah brought my attention back to another aspect of my profession. Everyone in this field is familiar with the way the popular media handle cosmetic surgery. The emphasis is consistently on the negative—"exploding boobs and exploding bums," as Sarah put it. There is rarely any discussion of the enormous benefits people experience, but in its place something that looks like moral indignation. What underlies this stuff?

As the years have gone on, I've had to contend with the fact that a significant body of opinion holds all cosmetic procedures to be, well, not wrong perhaps, but declassé. These are the people who strongly believe—and they will tell you so—that not only do they intend to "grow old gracefully" but they expect others to do the same. I am not a sociologist or psychologist and have made no systematic study of this phenomenon, but my impression is that these opponents of cosmetic procedures are also very often poorly disposed towards more common cosmetic practices such as applying make-up or dying one's hair. They judge these efforts to appear more youthful as vain and foolish, however much pleasure they may give the individuals who do apply lipstick or put a wash on their gray locks. They look askance at "inappropriate"—that is, youthful—clothing styles when worn by the middle-aged.

It's easy to recognize these attitudes as an ancient puritanical thread that has run through our culture and others for many centuries. It seems an indestructible part of human nature and may play an important role in regulating personal excesses. The operative word, however, is personal. Overall, the puritanical impulse is best served when applied to oneself rather than others. At its most essential, it can be grimly pleasure-denying—and denying pleasure, however satisfying for some, certainly doesn't suit all.

But there's more to the animus towards cosmetic medicine than a simple disapproval of pleasure. Look at the pages (and usually the covers) of the tabloids and see the ferocious coverage of "cosmetic surgery gone wrong."

Whether these lurid photographs are really what they purport to be or just aging actresses photographed in bad light, or recent proce-

But there's more to the animus towards cosmetic medicine than a simple disapproval of pleasure.

dures still healing, or actual uncorrected mistakes, is often unclear. What is clear is the sheer schadenfreude the writers—and presumably their readers—purport to take. Yet these publications cannot really be described as puritanical (often quite the opposite). So what drives this fierce approach?

"Envy," Sarah tells me. "It's like the headlines are saying, 'Look! Look at these people richer and more famous and better looking than you are! They thought they were so great because they could afford facelifts! Look at them now!' And people are reading this stuff and nodding and saying 'Yeah. Serves them right!'"

She smiles a bit sardonically.

"When I appear on television shows, I'll often find the hosts use the occasion to attack cosmetic surgery or even whip the audience into a frenzy of condemnation, like they did recently on The Doctors when they jumped on the fact that I've given my daughter—who's a model—a voucher for a future procedure. But afterwards, in the green room, these same hosts will often pump me for cosmetic surgery advice. Crikey."

But what about those vouchers, by the way? And the pole dancing?

Sarah laughs. "My daughter is a gymnast who loves Cirque du Soleil, your famous Canadian troupe that combines Chinese acrobatics and Western circus styles. That's the type of "pole dancing" Poppy does. And I get the gift certificates for free. I hope she can cash them in when she needs to for her education. My daughter would love to be a plastic surgeon and this will be money in the bank for her training if she decides to pursue it."

I myself had to express some sympathy for this sort of green-tinged sentiment that Sarah describes because many cosmetic procedures have been expensive in the past. But just as with other forms of new technology, these early adopters paid for the development of materials and techniques that are more and more available to everyone. We may have envied the people who could afford the first cell phones—$3000 apiece and as big as your arm—but they helped pay for the little devices that everyone of us carry today.

 "The fact is," Sarah Burge said, "good cosmetic surgery changes people's lives for the better."

"The fact is," Sarah Burge said, "good cosmetic surgery changes people's lives for the better. It's fine, people telling you that all beauty is inner beauty and that your funny nose, stuck-out ears, saggy eyelids or flabby arms shouldn't matter, but you know they do matter. When nobody could change these things, maybe resignation was the best attitude. But now we can change them. Why would someone try to stop you? It's like you want to visit Italy and somebody says, 'Don't do that. What's wrong with home? People weren't meant to fly.' Sorry. People *can* fly now. Don't hold them down."

My conversations with Sarah Burge were valuable in two respects. First, they confirmed how important is information when choosing a cosmetic practitioner—so important that it's called forth a new profession: the cosmetic surgery consultant, of which Sarah is an outstanding and highly visible example. Second, that there is a population of scolds ready to condemn others' efforts to find peace with their own appearance, and it often takes gumption to defy them.

I said goodbye to Sarah and her husband Tony with a sense that, for all the overheated publicity they'd received, they were making a contribution by opening eyes up everywhere and standing up proudly for cosmetic surgery clients. Maybe looking twenty years younger than one's age is not what everyone wants but it's good to know she's out there, still healthy and still carrying the standard for her convictions.

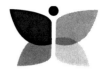

5 THE TOP TEN COSMETIC CONCERNS
(and who should address them for you)

I am not a cosmetic practitioner at the start of his career, nor at the end, but I've been doing this a long time, most of my adult life. One consequence is that I've got a strong sense of what concerns my patients most. I know the Internet is loaded with thousands of pages describing techniques and procedures, but most people are not in the business of studying medicine, and anyway, these pages are largely written by writers. That's why you're reading this book.

Of course, where you go with your concerns is partly dependant on what can be done to address them. That means I have to talk somewhat systematically about procedures. And because this chapter covers such a wide range of procedures—though it's by no means comprehensive—I must address a wide range of practitioners, from senior cosmetic surgeons with advanced medical degrees in related specialties to mall-front electrolysis clinics. I've tried as far as possible to provide some specific advice related to each concern, but it probably does no harm to review some things you should watch for in any office, big or small, long-established or advertising a just-opened introductory sale special. The now-familiar questions—How much training have they had? Are their certificates visible?—still apply and I urge you to use them when visiting prospective providers of cosmetic services.

One general comment. When cosmetic surgery began, it consisted of invasive procedures, all done under general anesthesia, with general anesthesia's inherent risks of death, disfigurement and downtime. When the surgery was done, the patient would have to hide away for an extended period of time—weeks, even months. There were bandages, drainage tubes and copious blood loss. Patients would require a prolonged recovery period. There was pain and what doctors call morbidity (in lay terms, "a diseased state"—in this case, a medically induced one).

Over twenty years ago, Botox® changed all that. Suddenly, people could be made to look better with little down time and the so-called promise of "non-invasive or minimally invasive procedures" became an expectation of modern cosmetic surgery. In time, more minimally invasive procedures associated with "a little" downtime and "a little" risk began to appear in numbers. This range of procedures should be thought of as a continuum, not discrete points on the scale. There is overlap. Invasive procedures, for example, are not nearly as invasive as they used to be. Indeed, many of them now border on minimally invasive. Some simple modern techniques can achieve results that would have challenged highly-trained experts forty years ago. I hope to guide you with my personal observations and comments, but your own homework is, as always, indispensable.

Where do I get my information? I host a radio show, *Inside Cosmetic Surgery Today*, on WebTalkRadio.net and a web-TV show at YourCosmeticDoctor.tv. In the course of producing these shows and covering the leading trends and procedures, I speak with dozens of world leaders in cosmetic surgery. I speak at conferences in Canada, the United States, Europe and the Middle East—especially Egypt—and so keep my finger on the pulse of exciting advances in the field.

I've distilled all that down to the Top Ten Cosmetic Concerns (and who should address them for you)—and the procedures to treat them. Here they are.

1. I'm unhappy with the appearance of my skin, especially my face.

"I look in the mirror and I don't recognize the face staring back at me."

For us human beings, the face is supremely important. It occupies the body's highest point and most of our sensory organs are concentrated there, immediately adjacent to our brains. We've become exquisitely skillful at recognizing and interpreting the faces of others, our foremost link to our fellow humanity. No wonder we take our faces seriously! But the face is also the most exposed part of the body and over the years of our lives, the most vulnerable to time's withering effects. When we consider cosmetic procedures, the face and neck are special too because their skin and the blood supply to that skin and the healing of that skin are different for the face than elsewhere on the body. Not surprisingly, different skills and procedures are necessary to deal with them. Let's look at some problems that are largely those of the face.

Acne

"I don't deserve this."

"I thought acne was a teenage thing. It's not."

"I didn't have acne as a kid. It started when I was 30. Why am I affected?"

"Why don't those TV products work?"

Many of the cosmetic issues that concern my patients are inherited characteristics or the results of aging. Not so with acne. It's important to recognize that *acne vulgaris* is a skin disease and not some simple reaction to a bad diet or lifestyle. The condition is characterized by red skin, blackheads

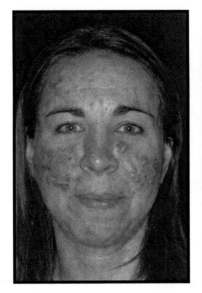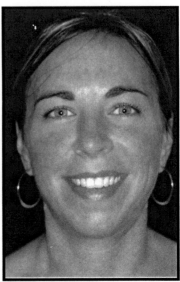

These before and after pictures of a pretty victim of severe acne demonstrate the enormous strides taken by modern cosmetic dermatology. Courtesy of C. Crutchfield.

and whiteheads, pinheads, pimples and sometimes scarring. Although it sometimes persists into adulthood past the age of twenty-five, and occasionally starts only in adulthood, acne is famously a disease of adolescence, one of the numerous torments associated with that period of life.

The causes of acne are complex and its treatment can also be complex. The immediate cause is blockage of the pores which in essence are tiny hair follicles. Associated with each pore is a tiny oil or sebaceous gland that becomes enlarged and clogged. That's acne. Under these conditions, the normally benign bacteria, *Propionibacterium acnes,* can multiply to produce inflammation that can be painful and leave lasting damage—scarring. Among the contributory factors are the hormonal imbalances of adolescence that can lead to enlargement of the follicles, infection by certain strains of bacteria and sometimes diet. Acne may also be associated with stress, although it's unclear which is the cause and which the effect. Diet, especially dairy products and foods with a high glycemic index (a measure of the effects of complex carbohydrates in food on blood sugar levels), has been implicated in acne. Hormones are also implicated, and exogenous hormones and various hormonal blocking agents can also be used to arrest acne in some women patients.

Serious cases of acne are best treated by a qualified dermatologist, a specialist who is familiar with the many drug options and their possible complications, or a doctor trained in the pathophysiology of this disease. Treatment may be with antibacterials, antibiotics, anti-inflammatories, hormones and hormonal blocking agents, lasers, light sources, dietary manipulation, surgery and a class of medications called retinoids that affect the follicle cells themselves.

Research into photo-therapy and photo-rejuvenation has led to an innovation in the treatment of acne that uses a high-intensity blue-violet light to precisely target porphyrins, substances on the skin that surface and ductal bacteria feed upon. These bacteria cause 90% of inflamed blemishes. The ClearLight Acne PhotoClearing System was the first non-drug treatment device approved by the FDA to treat moderate acne, followed more recently by Blue U. The companies that make these products claim that they produce results without the side effects of traditional acne treatments. I'm able to attest that, in my office, where we use a similar device—intense pulse light (IPL) with a headpiece attachment and the Blu U light therapy—we attain similar results.

These devices are an exciting addition to the acne armamentarium. Patients are exposed to the light after ALA (alpha leveulenic acid) is applied to the skin, often in 15-minute sessions. The treatment regimen consists of eight sessions over a period of four to eight weeks. A 2003 Reuters News Service report quotes Macrene Alexiades-Armenakas, MD, Ph.D., director of research at the Laser and Skin Surgery Center of New York, who is involved in clinical trials of the ClearLight device. He makes the important point that this relatively passive regimen is far more likely to be followed by teenagers. His initial results in 2003 suggested that, by four weeks, there was a "significant decrease" in acne bacterial counts. He cites one published study that showed a 60% reduction in *P. acnes* counts by eight weeks and an even larger decrease of 70% after two weeks of follow-up. The results appear to be sustained and no side effects have been observed.

We're often concerned with reducing the scarring that can be left by acne and the favoured tool is laser dermabrasion using a fractional CO_2 or a Er:YAG laser—or both. More recently, fractional and profractional therapy has been used. Further scar correction needs the full skill of a skilled doctor—often a dermatologist or a dermatological surgeon using injections, lasers, surgery, chemical peels, medications and everything in his "saddle bag" to get the best results. This is skilled work, normally carried out on the face, so you should entrust yourself only to a hands-on cosmetic doctor, surgically skilled and with considerable experience. But you must be realistic. Not even the best doctor can remove all traces of acne scarring.

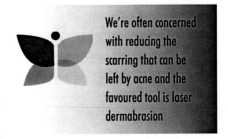

We're often concerned with reducing the scarring that can be left by acne and the favoured tool is laser dermabrasion

Personally, I have been treating acne and acne scarring for more than twenty years. While advances have helped with the treatment of acne and acne scarring, this still is one of the most difficult areas of cosmetic surgery. Recently, I saw a patient I treated 15 years ago. We used ALA and lasers to remove his acne. There are some minor scars there but he's not bothered by them. He's come in to thank me for what I had done. He is now attending college and his acne chapter is behind him. Similar stories have come from dozens of patients. I am thrilled and honored to have been involved in their care.

Sun Damage and Aging

*"I wish I'd known what the
sun could do to me much earlier.
When I was a kid I was told to
get out and get a tan."*

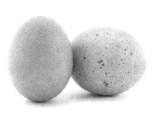

*"How can sun tan parlors be
in existence when they knowingly administer a proven
carcinogen?"*

*Y*ou have to be wondering why I'm heading this section with two different causes of skin damage. The fact is that the effects on our skin of the sun's ultraviolet rays take many forms, and one of those forms is the simple acceleration of the aging process. Many of my patients come to me for help in softening what seems to them to be the ravages of time but is actually the result of sun tanning over the years. The fact that this damage didn't show up when they were in their twenties doesn't exonerate the sun at all.

Having made that point I must also admit that, with or without the sun, the aging process goes on and cosmetic practitioners use many of the same procedures to deal with both. Hyper-pigmentation, fine wrinkles, yellowing, rough and/or dry skin, visible fine veins: whether the result of the sun, aging or both, they're a common cause of concern. A person can see these effects with a special ultraviolet B camera that

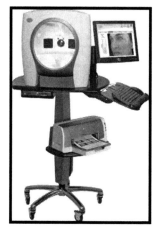

*The VISIA™ imaging
system allows us to
evaluate six aspects of skin
complexion health: visible
spots, pores, wrinkles,
evenness, porphyrins
and UV spots. The system
software enables the tracking
of treatment progress.*

clearly shows the damage "below the skin" that people cannot see on the surface. The effect is like shock therapy.

Let's look at the most important techniques and consider who is best suited to apply them.

Cosmetics and Cosmeceuticals

"There is such a plethora of products, I really don't know what to choose."

"I used to go to the drug store or department store to buy products. Not any longer. I wouldn't trust my skin to a cosmetic salesperson named Bambi."

At first blush (as it were) you might think it strange that a book on cosmetic surgery would have a section on cosmetics. Yet cosmetic agents have an important role in cosmetic medicine because they help a doctor do what cosmetic surgery cannot do alone. Cosmetics enhance and prolong the results of cosmetic surgeries. The late Albert Kligman, professor emeritus of the University of Pennsylvania and co-developer of Retin A, coined the term "cosmeceutical" twenty-five years ago to describe the role cosmetics were assuming by literally combining "cosmetics" and "pharmaceuticals."

In fact cosmetics today probably do a great deal more than cosmetic companies are willing to admit, because if the companies were to demonstrate that their products actively affected change in the skin, they might find them reclassified as "drugs" and subject to more strenuous regulation. Regardless, the new generation of cosmetic products are much different from those of a few decades ago. Back then, their primary effect was preventing the skin from losing water; in other words, these mixtures of oil and water were "moisturizers." Now cosmetics have active ingredients that actively affect how skin looks and behaves. It's beyond the scope of this book to go into greater depth about the activity of cosmeceuticals, but I can tell you that, from my personal observations, the best of these products can be very effective in correcting acne, sun damage, hyperpigmentation, fine wrinkles, yellowing (sallowness), rough texture and dryness. A good cosmetic doctor should be able to advise you as to what product can help your particular condition. He should take into account your unique characteristics and use his knowledge to prescribe appropriate cosmetics for you, just as he would prescribe medication.

Personally, I believe cosmetics and cosmeceuticals are the basis on which to build therapeutics of the skin. You can't have a beautiful face without beautiful skin. And you can't have beautiful skin without properly used cosmetics and cosmeceuticals.

Can you trust the poorly educated commission salesman at the cosmetic counter of your pharmacy or department store to adminster advice on these agents? I think you know the answer.

Low-Level Laser Therapy (LLLT)

Can low-energy light sources "turn on" the healing mechanism of the skin?

Low-level laser light therapy (LLLT), which employs lasers, and deep-penetrating light therapy (DPLT), which employs light-emitting diodes (LEDs), has been used for some years to relieve pain and inflammation in physical therapy and occupational medicine, mainly for sports injuries. It has been somewhat controversial but widely practiced. Its employment in cosmetic medicine began in 2004, with the publication of a paper describing a system that used light-emitting diodes (LED) therapy to lessen the effects of photoaging. The majority of patients demonstrated improvement in fine wrinkles around the eyes, reduction in Fitzpatrick photoaging classification, improvement in global skin texture and background erythema and pigmentation. No side effects were noted. Whether based on lasers or LEDs, this procedure regulates cell activity using light sources without any heat effect. Further studies have shown skin textural improvement accompanied by increased collagen deposition.

As with every minimally invasive procedure, there are those who question whether this modality works. The reason is that the results are subtle and hard to quantify. But with repeat treatments, I've found that most patients note significant difference in their skin.

How many treatments are necessary to get results? Most experts would say about twenty, done twice weekly.

How much training is required to operate this equipment? A trick question: these units are so idiot-proof, a trained chimpanzee can operate one.

How effective? On a scale of one to ten, one being minimal results, ten being awesome results, I would rate LLT as a 3 or a 5.

From Dermabrasion and Microdermabrasion to Lasers

In the last three decades, there has been an explosion of interest in this area. We now have hugely effective tools to help rejuvenate the skin.

Not surprisingly, most damage to the skin occurs on the surface and in the upper layers of the skin. Cosmetic doctors recognized the problem early on and developed procedures to remove fine wrinkles, superficial skin growths, shallow scars, pigment changes in the skin and other skin problems. The earliest and most basic of these techniques involved sanding away the top layer of skin using a fast revolving wire brush or diamond wheel, a technique termed "ablative resurfacing," much like an auto mechanic would do when he was doing body work on a vehicle. It allows new skin to grow and is most often used to treat acne scars and wrinkles around the mouth. This was technically difficult to do, so difficult in fact, that this has largely been replaced by lasers and a technique known as laser abrasion. In this technique, highly tuned CO_2 and erbium lasers literally evaporate the top layers of the skin. More recently, fractional resurfacing and

profractional resurfacing does something similar by putting bo-
luses of energy into the skin through tiny holes.

Microdermabrasion, using a jet of fine grit—often inert crystals of aluminum oxide—and removing them with a vacuum, was
first used in the 1980s as a less invasive form of dermabrasion. It
has evolved rapidly since: a newer version accomplishes the same
result without crystals, using only a diamond or bristle tip. These
procedures may be followed by cream and cosmeceutical applications that enhance the abrasive's penetration into skin and in turn
enhance the effectiveness of skin care products. There is little or
no downtime.

Most recently, there has been a marriage of laser abrasions,
profractional and fractional resurfacing with other modalities.
One is the use of IPLs—intense pulsed lights. These light sources also treat red and brown lesions in the skin. I'll cover this later.

Another is the application of PRP or platelet rich plasma, blood
plasma that has been enriched with platelets. As a concentrated
source of autologous platelets— platelets drawn from the patient's
own blood—PRP contains various growth factors and other cytokines that stimulate healing of bone and soft tissue and "call in"
stem cells to enhance that healing. Platelet rich plasma is either
injected into the skin or applied to the surface of the skin after
therapy. Combined with fractional and profractional resurfacing,
it has an augmenting effect. I recently covered the scientific aspects of this at a Rxderm conference in Austin and at Sharm Derma, the major dermatology conference in the Middle East.

The degree of difficulty in using abrasive techniques varies from
miniscule for microdermabrasion to horrendous for dermabrasion
and laser abrasion. Most procedures are in between. For simple
procedures like microdermabrasion, an adequately trained esthetician can probably handle it. For fractional and profractional resurfacing, a well trained laser technician should be up to the job.
But when you get onto the deeper, more aggressive procedures,
treatments should be done by a doctor—and not just any doctor

but the best available in the community.

The costs will vary according to how difficult the procedure is to do and to how well trained the doctor is. You tend to pay for what you get.

With simple procedures, there is no downtime, but as you get into the deeper, more invasive procedures, the downtime may be considerable. For example, fractional or pro-fractional resurfacing has one to four days of downtime. With dermabrasion and laser abrasion, initial healing is in one to two weeks and the residual erythema (redness) may take months to abate. The use of PRP has diminished this period.

Light and Very Light Chemical Peels

There are peelers and healers. The two work together like hand and glove.

Like dermabrasion, chemical peeling is a skin resurfacing procedure but one that uses a chemical solution to remove the top layers of the skin, allowing new skin to grow. Chemical peels are available in various strengths, with the strongest removing more skin, posing greater chances of complications—and potentially greater benefits. The mildest produce little or no downtime but require repeated use to get results. The deepest peels often require as long as three to four weeks for a full recovery and there are risks associated with removing this much tissue, infection being the most serious.

Personally, I have found a series of low-strength chemical peels to be equivalent to a medium-strength peel, with the patient receiving the benefits with little or no downtime.

A technician can do light peels but heavier peels require a qualified cosmetic doctor and in some cases an anesthetist. A weekend course is not nearly enough, even for simple peels. I myself am still constantly learning after twenty-plus years in practice. You should know all costs and options beforehand, and while you're at it, your doctor should discuss the possibility of complications.

Every doctor experiences complications and should be able to put them in perspective for you.

Fractional, Non-ablative Laser Resurfacing and Non-Fractional, Ablative Resurfacing

ℒasers can be wonderful tools. In no area of cosmetic medicine has there been a more dramatic evolution in our understanding of our technology. Lasers can also be entirely ineffective. Believe me, at least half my grey hairs can be attributed to lasers. Never assume that just because a clinic offers laser treatment, that the lasers are the right kind or in the right hands. I've purchased lasers that I ultimately concluded were useless. It's sometimes said that, for patients, the word "laser" means Lots of Applications of Sexy Exciting Resources. To a doctor who has been around cosmetic circles as long as I have, it means Lots of Aggravation by Expensive Sophisticated Resources. When you're considering a laser procedure, your general investigation of a prospective practitioner should include some questions about the actual equipment. If you discover the make and model, you can ask other doctors for their opinion and exploit the Internet to get more information.

Laser resurfacing is typically used to remove or improve the appearance of fine wrinkles, shallow scars (from acne, surgery, or trauma), tattoos and other skin defects. The technology is constantly changing as researchers search for improvements and again, lasers are no guarantee of a happy outcome. So-called fractional resurfacing using lasers, now very widely used, employ heat induced by laser light to put tiny holes in the upper layers of the skin. Fractional resurfacing has largely replaced ablative resurfacing because true ablative resurfacing was a substantial procedure with considerable downtime required to heal the wounds. In fractional resurfacing, columns of energy are put deep into the skin and the surface of the skin remains relatively undisturbed. The result is usually little downtime and good to great results. Erbium lasers were the first lasers that were fractionated and they penetrated slightly into the upper layer of the skin, known as the dermis. CO_2 laser resurfacing goes deeper, affecting the part of the skin known as the dermis, causing new skin and collagen to grow and so improving results.

Recently I've been using a deep resurfacing tool known as the SCAAR (or "synergistic coagulation and ablation for advanced resurfacing") laser to treat severe burn scars. This new technology penetrates deeply. I'm in constant communication with Matteo Tretti Clementon and Chad Hivnor, some of the pioneers in this area, as we establish the protocols necessary for optimal scar rejuvenation. the addition of platelet-rich plasma has enhanced healing times and new lasers such as the SCAAR laser by Lumenis have further enhanced results by combining penetrance with coagulation and ablation.

The experience required to perform these laser procedures is difficult to quantify. I actually have my technician do our fractional erbium resurfacing, but she was trained by me and performed a hundred under my supervision before I felt her to be competent. For CO_2 fractional resurfacing, I believe this must be done by a doctor who has had extensive training and handled at least dozens of cases. And for ablative resurfacing, you should consider only doctors who've handled hundreds of cases. It's such doctors' communications with the world's experts that is key to staying abreast of the most

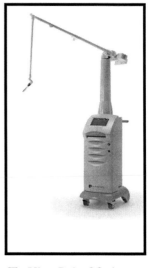

The Ultra Pulse CO_2 has many uses. It can be used for facial resurfacing, actinic keratoses, basal cell carcinoma, acne scars, burn debridement and surgical scars. The ActiveFX option allows superficial fractional ablation for fine lines, uneven texture, dyschromia and actinic keratosis.

advancing technology.

As to price, be wary of one that seems too low. Laser procedures may vary from perhaps $500 to thousands of dollars, based on what needs to be done. Laser resurfacing clearly has several complex components. Anesthesia is often required and the doctor must choose the proper procedure.

And as to results, well, they'll vary with the depth, the type of laser, the penetration and whether ablative or fractional resurfacing is used and adjuvant procedures done. One thing though is certain: 100% resolution of scars, aging and sun damage cannot be achieved. I like to say that 50-80% is reasonable. Since I have been practicing cosmetic surgery, lasers have evolved significantly, but remember, they remain instruments—mere tools—that may both help and harm. Be respectful and wary of them. They are not magic devices like Luke Skywalker's "light sabre."

ALA/PDT/Blue and Red Light

This class of procedure, called "photodynamic therapy" or "photo-activated chemotherapy" is an emerging therapy and essentially another type of targeted destruction of unwanted tissue—resurfacing, in other words. In its cosmetic applications, it is generally regarded as minimally invasive and minimally toxic. It employs a photoactive chemical (ALA) applied to the skin and then activated by a light source such as a laser or a blue light, with the result that highly reactive oxygen molecules are created. These so-called "free radicals" are what actually kill the unwanted cells.

The difficulty in this procedure is that the stratum corneum, the top layer of the skin, prevents the ALA from penetrating, and without penetration, the ALA just won't work. To achieve the penetration, a thorough microdermabrasion or acetone treatment needs to be accomplished and the ALA left on for a proper length of time in order to "incubate." Such a tricky protocol is best done under the supervision of a medical professional. Expect to pay about $400 to $1,000 per session.

I have had tremendous success with this modality and more than a few failures, mainly in the way of burns. Thankfully, I have seen relatively few long lasting scars. Have your doctor compare the merits of this procedure with others he or she offers.

Photorejuvenation: Intense Pulsed Light (IPL) and Broad Band Light (BBL)

Like the other light therapies we've already discussed, IPL has found wide application in the treatment of damaged skin. Introduced to the market about a decade ago as an alternative to lasers, IPL procedures can produce similar results at a lower cost. Instead of laser light or photoactive chemicals, IPL employs a series of intense pulses of light to improve the appearance of rosacea, flushing, broken capillaries, hirsutism (excessive hair), sun-damaged skin, age spots, skin texture and photo-aging. To combat burning, the devices are equipped with dynamic cooling mechanisms.

Although this procedure may sound simple, it's not. I've seen tremendous burns caused by unqualified practitioners. The typical training offered by the providing companies is a day-long session. Some colleges offer a week's orientation to lasers and IPLs. Again, in my opinion, this is inadequate. It takes weeks of hands-on training under a IPL expert—probably 50 to 100 procedures—to achieve sufficient mastery of this tool. That's why the most important question you should ask is, "Where did you train and how many cases have you done?" these machines, like lasers, are only as safe and effective as the operator.

If you opt for IPL therapy, expect to spend several hundred to several thousand dollars depending on the work that needs to be done.

Botox

Not all effective treatments of the skin rely on the destruction of surface tissue. All wrinkles, for example, cannot be abraded away.

One of the most famous of all cosmetic procedures and the

one that truly remade modern cosmetic surgery, is the use of the botulinum toxin injected into facial muscles to block the nerve signals that tell the muscle to contract. This temporarily—a few months usually—weakens the muscle and has the effect of smoothing wrinkles in the skin.

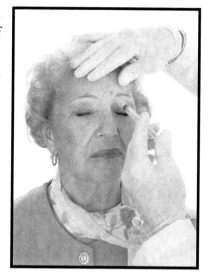

Like some other techniques, Botox was originally used as a solution to one problem but has been adapted to others. Recently I interviewed one of these innovators, Dr. Woffles Wu of Singapore, on my radio show *Inside Cosmetic Surgery Today*. Wu is using Botox for smoothing the skin, lifting the brow, decreasing skin oiliness, shrinking large pores, acne, keloids, hypertrophic scars and shaping the lower face by decreasing the size of hypertrophic masseter muscles. We may see his techniques become more widely used.

Although Botox appears to be very safe, recent reports of side effects of large dose Botox used in medical conditions has cast a cloud on Botox use. Personally, I believe these alarms are overstated. The worst complication I've seen is the temporary weakening of muscle around the eyes when Botox affects unintended muscles.

The best uses in my opinion is in rejuvenation of the upper face used in combination with fillers such as those we'll discuss later in this chapter.

There is a lot of controversy as to the best Botox dilution and dosage for different areas. However, the injection technique is simple provided the practitioner pays attention to detail. That's probably why Dr. Alastair Carruthers, one of the co-founders of the cosmetic use of Botox, says, "Close is close enough for horse-shoes, hand grenades, and Botox."

For easy Botox cases, minimal training such as a day-long course is usually sufficient. However, to truly understand the use of this agent, a practitioner must understand fillers, lasers, and cosmetic correction. Personally, I would choose the most quali-fied person in your area. Remember to ask if your doctor teach-es others on this procedure, since experienced experts tend to become teachers of others. And it won't hurt to find out if your doctor has spoken on Botox at international symposia, or writ-ten about it or appeared on recognized broadcast programs to discuss Botox. The more experienced hands you're in, the better hands you're in.

In general, expect to pay around $500 for each area treated. There has been a trend towards low-cost Botox, charged by the unit. I personally strongly discourage you from these seductive promotions. Low-cost Botox tempts practitioners to cut corners and when they do so, complications arise.

I recently attended a meeting of the American Academy of Dermatology at which Jean and Alistair Carruthers were pre-sented with lifetime achievement awards for dermatology. Yet, when they began using Botox for cosmetic reasons in the late 1980s, they were vilified by the press. What in the world were dermatologists doing using one of the world's deadliest poison's to treat wrinkles? Times have changed and Botox has proven it-self a valuable part of cosmetic medicine.

Ulthera, Thermage and Other Tissue-Tightening Technologies

These procedures use heat in the form of high-intensity ultrasound waves, radio waves or infrared light to tighten and to a certain extent lift the skin of the face and neck without surgery. Thermage and related technologies protect the skin surface with a cooling action while heating the deep layers underneath. The aim is to cause immediate collagen contraction

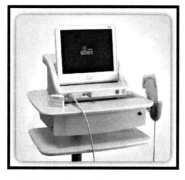

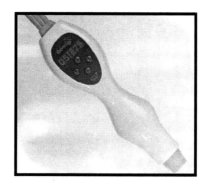

Ulthera: Focused ultrasound for skin therapy

Solta Thermage: skin tightening using radio frequency waves

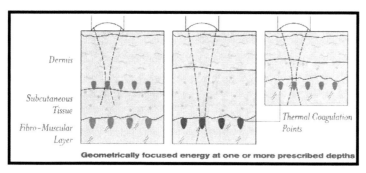

Ulthera: The Principle: focused energy at depth

followed by new collagen production.

Can a non-invasive therapy actually lift and tighten the skin? I find that patients continue to show improvement at least six months after treatment. For a non-invasive technology, the results have truly been amazing.

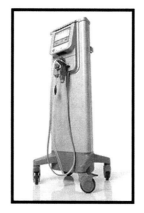

The Thermage Unit

2. As I grow older, my face is sagging, creasing and hollowing. I am 70 but I feel 50 so why should I look 70?

Some evidence of aging is beyond resurfacing and too much even for Botox and thermage. Here we enter the realm formerly ruled by the face lift and other serious surgical interventions, but now shared with less-invasive lifts and fillers. This is truly the "new cosmetic surgery."

Thread Lifts

Sometimes referred to as "aptos threads," this ingenious technique employs specially-designed barbed polypropylene threads, strongly anchored to the dermis, that are tugged up to lift and suspend the skin and subcutaneous fat. The result is a visible yet subtle facial rejuvenation such as that achieved through a modest facelift. There are issues of maintenance, however, since the tiny barbs can slip down with time and when this occurs the threads must be surgically removed and reinserted. Nonetheless, I've seen threads give results for up to 10 years.

During the recession of 2008, the company making the threadlift materials left the cosmetic surgery market. I predict these threads will re-emerge at some point in the future.

Fillers

If you have thin lips or deep creases anywhere on your face or neck, there are many exciting advances in cosmetic surgery to help you. Known as "fillers," they fill in wrinkles, creases and depressed scars. After the first-developed filler, bovine-derived collagen, proved to have limitations, many different filler options

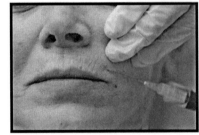

have come to the forefront over the last few years.

NASHA ("non-animal stabilized hyaluronic acid"), Restylane®, Teosyl® and Juvederm® are well-known examples based on hyaluronic acid. Because natural hyaluronic acid wouldn't last long (the body has enzymes that degrade it), these products are made from a stabilized variety that degrades slowly, and when it degrades, traps more water, maintaining its correction for an average of nine months in most patients.

In my experience, patients love their results. I predict filler use will escalate, especially in combination therapies.

PRP (Vampire Lift, Selphyl, Platelet Rich Plasma)

*D*espite the name, this is not a scalpel technique but a filler. Platelets and other components in human blood migrate to a site of injury and are known to release a variety of factors that respond to that injury and promote healing. By concentrating platelets at the site of injury, physicians have the potential to enhance the body's natural capacity for healing.

PRP takes a patient's own plasma and combines it with an activating agent. The surgeon puts the mixture under the skin. The result is a new filling agent which stimulates the creation of endogenous (that is, internally generated) collagen and recruits stem cell migration to an area. The technique beautifies the skin and has proven very useful in peri-ocular rejuvenation.

Charles Crutchfield and I recently wrote an article on PRP for the "Online Dermatology Journal" and I presented on the technique—called "Lenvisage"—at the Rxderm conference in Austin, Texas. Because this material forms a masting such that lesser amounts of other fillers are necessary, I envisage its widespread use as a filler-sparing agent.

The "Liquid Facelift"

A liquid facelift employs the use of a combination of techniques: the injection of platelet-rich plasma and botulinum A, with the

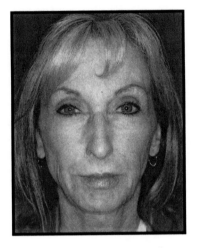 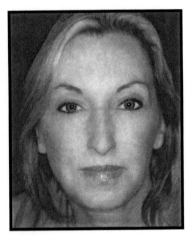

The "liquid facelift" points the way to the future of cosmetic medicine: minimally invasive techniques, often in combination, that achieve results once only associated with serious surgery.

application of hyaluronic acid, alpha hydroxyl peels, and sometimes laser rejuvenation.

The Stem Cell Lift

As you might have guessed from PRP, above, stem cells—basically cells that haven't yet decided what to be when they grow up—have recently become all the rage in medicine, with numerous applications being explored. As Ron Moy, former president of the American Academy of Dermatology, testified in our earlier interview on this book, cosmetic medicine is no exception. Stem cells may now be harvested from the donor's own fat and injected with the donor's own fat in appropriate sites, where they act as more natural and better-bonded filler that more permanently and effectively regenerates and revitalizes tissues. This is cutting-edge medicine, but watch for rapid development if results fulfill the present promise.

I recently interviewed Dr. Nathan Newman

of Beverly Hills California, an expert in the stem cell lift and an early pioneer in this treatment.

http://webtalkradio.net/internet-talk-radio/2012/02/20/inside-cosmetic-surgery-today-%E2%80%93-using-our-stem-cells-to-repair-our-bodies-dr-lycka-dr-newman/

The Face Lift

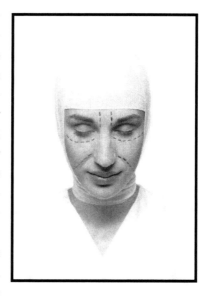

In this classic surgical procedure, the surgeon literally lifts the skin off the face so that the structures beneath the skin (the superficial musculoaponeurotic system or SMAS) can be tightened and the skin smoothed back over the face. A facelift is perhaps the most famous and definitely the most comprehensive approach to treating the wrinkles and sagging of the face and the neck that are caused by age. It also requires the highest degree of expertise on the part of the surgeon.

Traditionally, the facelift was the primary tool for treating the aging face. But it became evident that sagging or drooping was only part of the clinical spectrum of aging. Two other components—decay and deflation—also needed to be addressed for optimal results. When this realization came about, the whole paradigm for treating the face changed. Fillers replaced the deflation; lasers, IPLs, chemical peels, cosmeceuticals and Botox corrected the decay. It became apparent that in many cases, facelifts could be delayed or even omitted by concentrating on these elements.

When drooping is the primary component in a face's decline, nothing works as well as a facelift. The problem is that the procedure has been associated with significant downtime and morbidity, plus side effects including nerve damage and infection. How did modern cosmetic science deal with these factors? Through invention.

Dr. Davis Nguyen invented the Fibrin Face Lift, a modification of the facelift lift using fibrin, which improves and enhances the results and decreases downtime. You can listen to Dr. Nguyen at http://webtalkradio.net/internet-talk-radio/2011/08/20/inside-cosmetic-surgery-today-%E2%80%93-what-you-need-to-know-about-the-fibrin-facelift/

Meanwhile, neck lifts are being made easier by a new procedure known as the iGuide or the "trampoline lift." I recently discussed this breakthrough with Dr. Michelle Yagoda, a New York-based plastic surgeon who had been doing it for over a year at the time. She explained how this lift does not involve the incisions that are the hallmark of conventional lifts developed to improve the sagging neck. Instead, liposuction is followed by the use of a blunt minimally-invasive rod that threads a suture beneath the skin of the neck under the jawline. When the suture is tightened the neck is lifted.

As this book was going to press, Dr. Gregory Mueller, developer of the iGuide technique—termed a "trampoline platysmaplasty"—could be seen demonstrating it on various YouTube videos.

Facelifts are here to stay. What will change is that they will become less invasive with even less downtime for patients. Non-invasive lifting techniques such as Ulthera and iGuide have already demonstrated this.

The Brow Lift

*J*ust as faces fall, so do brows. Surgeons perform brow lifts using one of two procedures. In the classic browlift, an incision is made from ear to ear but above the hairline. In the endoscopic lift, a tiny camera is inserted under the skin through one incision and small surgical tools are inserted through another small incision. In both techniques, the surgeon then manipulates tissues to eliminate deep brow wrinkles and frown lines. The endoscopic lift also employs tiny anchors to hold tissues in new positions.

It should go without saying that brow lifts, like facelifts—they really are lifts of the face above the eyes—call for skill and experience on the surgeon's part. Botox, fillers, lasers and thread lifts have all been used to lift the brow non-surgically with less downtime. Brow lifts are still necessary, though, as I discussed recently with Dr Kolb on *Inside Cosmetic Surgery Today*.

The Eye Lift

*I*f we all live long enough, almost everyone will need their eye lids lifted. That's because there is a natural tendency for eyelids to droop and become baggy with time. Called blepharoplasty, this surgical procedure reshapes eyelids to remove bagginess and tightens loose skin around the eyelids, but doesn't remove fine wrinkle lines. It employs precise techniques to remove extra tissue and sew the remaining tissue back together. An eyelift is a significant procedure with 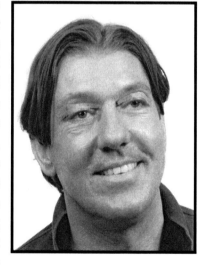 a high degree of patient satisfaction. Recently, the trend has been to be more conservative on the lower eyelid to avoid a "skeletized" look. Fillers, PRP and Botox have all proved useful adjuncts.

3. I have areas of stubborn fat that I can't get rid of and/or I'm otherwise unhappy with the shape of my body.

I should make it clear that body sculpting—in particular liposuction (also known as suction lipectomy or suction lipolysis)—has been my cosmetic specialty for much of my career. I encountered it early, adopted it early and have kept abreast of its continuous development. I have watched and participated in that development with the greatest satisfaction, since body sculpting, at its successful best, is one of cosmetic surgery's most satisfying procedures for patients. As a specialist in this area, I hear a lot of stories from patients who are battling private anguish about body shape.

> "I'm a police officer, so I keep in shape. But I hate going to the gym and having guys say stuff like, "Buy a bra, Bob." I'm tough as nails but I hate my breasts. Men's boobs "moobs"—yech!"

> "I'm a hairstylist. I hate going to work because my clients rub against my belly when I cut their hair. You can rub the Buddha's belly but not mine."

> "I tried so hard to make my marriage work with an ex who called me fat and ugly. So when I got my settlement, I knew the first thing I was going to do was get liposuction. I really wanted to make his new girl friend jealous and I knew I could look better than her."

> "It really is embarrassing. I try to eat properly and exercise but I don't see results."

> "I'm a professional trainer. I work out with my clients every day, sometimes twelve hours a day. But as I work out, my fat shows more. I really have "abs of steel" under the fat. They just don't show."

"I'm 78 years old but feel 20. I've outlived three husbands. You know what they say: 'Just because there is snow on the roof doesn't mean there's no fire in the furnace.' It's now my turn. I deserve to look good when I go to the symphony. I want to look the way I feel."

"I could keep my weight off until I injured my knee and couldn't exercise any more. The inches just came on."

"I wish I could turn back the clock and wear that little black dress again!"

Let's look at the techniques that offer solutions to the problems.

Liposuction (Lipoplasty, Suction Lipolysis)

Liposuction is the removal of stubborn excess fat from the body using a suction apparatus and cannulas—small, thin, blunt-tipped tubes. In traditional liposuction, the cannulas are inserted through tiny incisions in the skin. Fat is suctioned out through the cannulas as the doctor moves the cannula around under the skin to target specific fat deposits. There has been a continuous series of advances in liposuction techniques—tumescent liposuction, power-assisted liposuction, laser lipolysis and ultrasound-assisted liposuction. I describe them further below and in some detail in my earlier book, *SkinWorks*, but here are a few highlights.

Tumescent Liposuction

Tumescent liposuction was for years considered the safest and most effective liposuction technique, with the quickest recovery time. In tumescent liposuction, a large amount of an anesthetic solution containing lidocaine and epinephrine is injected into the fatty tissue before traditional liposuction is performed. The solution makes the fat expand and become firmer, which allows the cannula to move more smoothly under the skin. It also causes the blood vessels to shrink temporarily (vasoconstriction), which greatly reduces blood loss during the procedure.

Laser-Assisted Liposuction (laser lipolysis, SmartLipo®ʺ Thin Lipo)

The benefits of laser-assisted liposuction are that the laser melts the fat before suctioning is done, thus decreasing trauma. As a bonus it also contracts loose skin. The end result for the patient is less downtime and improved results.

Ultrasonic Lipolysis

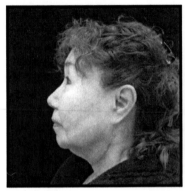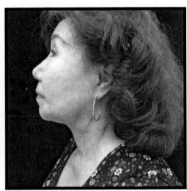

"Smart laser liposuction" is a technical advance that has permitted the application of liposuction to ever more refined cosmetic effects.

Ultrasonic lypolysis is a technique using focused ultrasound to remove fat cells, which are then vacuumed away as in other types of liposuction. Approved in many countries, it has yielded good to very good results in some hands, not so good in others. Your careful investigation of prospective surgeons is key to your satisfaction.

Liposuction: A Final Word

Since its introduction in the 1980s, liposuction has been made more effective and safer with the invention of the "tumescent" technique that involves the injection of fluid containing local anaesthetics, the ultrasonic-assisted and external ultrasonic techniques, and the "laser lypolysis" techniques that effectively dissolve the fat before it is suctioned away. These are all relatively recent developments and many surgeons and patients have contributed to the relatively safe and highly effective procedure performed today. We owe much to them and to the tools they helped develop. Yet through all of this one huge factor overwhelms all others: the skill and experience of the surgeon who is actually standing over the operating table. Liposuction is not a procedure ca-

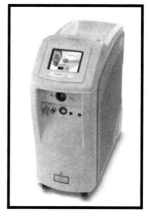

A laser lipolysis unit. No matter how sophisticated, advanced cosmetic tools are only as good as the hands that guide them.

sually taught to office assistants. It is a hand-and-eye skill acquired through patient learning and exercised by an accomplished surgeon.

Liposuction is not for everyone. It is no substitute for a good diet and a healthy exercise regimen. But many people whose lifestyles are beyond reproach are still left with stubborn areas of fat. They inherited them, to be blunt. As in the patients' stories I recounted earlier, these are the right folks for liposuction. They should have chosen their parents more wisely.

How do you find the right liposuction surgeon? By applying every piece of advice in this book. Because, aside from the facelift, few procedures require more skill or are more invasive.

By now you'll be familiar with the sorts of questions you should ask. But since this is an area I know so well, let me list some again.

- ♦ How long have you been doing liposuction surgery?
- ♦ What type of liposuction do you do?
- ♦ What can I expect?

- Can I talk to someone who's had it done?
- What do we do if I'm not satisfied?
- What happens if I have an unforeseen complication?
- How many cases have you done?
- What is your satisfaction rate"

And a final question you should ask *yourself*: Is this doctor busy? A busy doctor is busy for a reason.

Other Body Sculpting Technologies

*L*iposuction does not have the field to itself. Because it is a moderately invasive surgical technique, it has had its share of complications in the past and is still approached with trepidation by some patients. Clearly, procedures that would be less invasive but still effective, stand to make a strong appeal. This is a development parallel to the revolutionary changes in facial surgery—techniques such as the threads and various fillers—that represent a move down a less risky road towards less spectacular results.

Thermal Lipolysis (Lyposonix)

*T*his new technique heats the fat compartment from the outside using high intensity focused ultrasound. The fat is claimed to literally "melt away"—not the large volumes that liposuction is capable of removing, but enough to make a significant difference in appearance. It's too soon to line up with definite claims for this approach, but it is essentially non-surgical and therefore non-invasive. Like so many techniques, it is a work in progress.

Low Energy Lasers (Lapex 2000, Zerona)

*R*ather like thermal lipolysis, these machines target fat cells from outside the body and make them leaky so that the body absorbs the fat. They work temporarily, and require some degree of maintenance therapies.

Mesotherapy (LipoDissolve, Injection Lipolysis)

Mesotherapy employs medications that break down the fat-cell membrane and let the fat escape the cell. It is a simpler, less invasive technique than liposuction—and for some purposes more effective. The medications are injected into the mesoderm—the middle (fat) layer of the skin. Once broken down, the displaced fat enters the bloodstream, where it is either burned as energy or excreted. An improved form of mesotherapy, called "lipodissolve," uses more effective medications.

Like many things, mesotherapy started in other areas of medicine. Dr. Michel Pistor was among the first to use it to treat sports injuries. It evolved to where it was used in cosmetic surgery to treat unwanted fat deposits, cellulite and rejuvenate the skin.

There's no doubt that mesotherapy is somewhat controversial and its effectiveness hasn't been established by gold-standard clinical trials. However, the most serious accusations appear to arise from improper use and unsafe chemical agents. It is a useful technique for treating small areas of fat and some cases of cellulite. It certainly can be painful and there is the possible side effect of edema. Nonetheless, I use it in my practice and I believe it has its rightful place in any cosmetic doctor's armentarium.

CoolSculpting (Cryolipolysis)

CoolSculpting™ (or more formally, cryolipolysis) was developed by Zeltiq Aesthetics, Inc., a medical device company based in Pleasanton, California and established in 2005. Cryolipolysis was created by Drs. R. Rox Anderson and Dieter Manstein of Harvard Medical School and the Wellman Center for Photomedicine at Massachusetts General Hospital in Boston, MA. Their initial work, first published in the peer-reviewed professional journal *Lasers in Surgery and Medicine*, proved that subcutaneous fat cells are naturally more vulnerable to the effects of cold than are skin, nerve and muscle tissues and that it is possible to trigger natural cell death (apoptosis) by delivering cooling through the skin's surface. So-called "precise energy extraction" or "selective cryolipolysis" is basically cold used to injure only fat cells without damaging the overlying skin. It is postulated that the mechanisms at work include crystallization of lipids within fat cells and the technique's effectiveness appears to be limited to discrete fat bulges.

This is a very new procedure, not as yet widely available. Nonetheless, keep an eye on cryolipolysis. Such relatively non-invasive approaches seem to be the future. I recently lectured on this topic at MSR 2000 in Sharm El Sheikh, Egypt. I also interviewed Charles Crutchfield on CoolSculpting.

http://webtalkradio.net/2011/07/25/inside-cosmetic-surgery-today-coolscuplting-can-you-really-remove-fat-by-freezing

Extrinsic Ultrasonic Lipolysis (Ultrashape)

Ultrashape uses focused ultrasound to target small areas of fat. Ariel Brentrich of Montreal is perhaps the best known user of this modality. The difficulty lies in achieving reproducible results as the practitioner's technique is paramount in this procedure

After trying this technique in my clinic for a few months, I decided it was not for me.

Endermologie (also Veloshape)

The endermologie procedure was invented in France in the mid 1980s by Louis Paul Guitay, a French engineer who was receiving manual physical therapy to soften contracted scars he was left with after an accident. To standardize and facilitate the work of the therapist, he developed a mechanical device based on the principles of manual skin rolling. It powered a computer driven handheld massaging head that delivered intermittent suction and rolling to the area being treated as well as to the sub-adjacent soft tissue. Subsequently, it was found to diminish cellulite and that's where it really became popular. I was introduced to this technique by the late Jeffrey Arenswald of Las Vegas, Nevada. It uses a suction-assisted massage to help reduce cellulite and recontour the body. Whatever its mechanism, it's often a useful adjunct to liposuction because it can reduce the irregularities sometimes left by that procedure. In my view, endermologie has a place in the temporary and longer-term treatment of cellulite, but to achieve the best results, maintenance is necessary.

Breast Surgery

*B*reast surgeries are for the benefit of three patient types:
♦ those who want larger breasts
♦ those who want their aging breasts to look better
♦ those who want smaller breasts

Breast Augmentation

*B*reast augmentation and the other procedures in this section return us to the realm of invasive surgical intervention. In the minds of many, these procedures seem less daunting than the famous facelift and which I attribute to the huge emphasis we put on the face. These are, however, serious operations to be undertaken after careful consultation with an experienced professional.

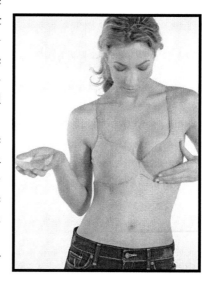

Dr. D. K. Hoffman of the San Francisco Bay area is a specialist in breast augmentation surgery. These are the sorts of things he hears from patients regularly:
♦ "I kept waiting for my

breasts to grow and they never did!"
♦ "I want to feel like a woman."
♦ "I want to be able to wear cute tops."
♦ "I want to wear a swim suit and look good in it."
♦ "I nursed my children and I just want my breasts to look like they used to."
♦ "I want to feel more confident."

Breast implants (also known as breast enlargement or augmentation) are saline- or silicone-filled bags slid in between the breast tissue and the chest muscles, or between the chest muscles and the chest wall. The same implant procedures, using bags filled with saline or silicone, are also being used to augment buttocks and even the male chest.

On Inside Cosmetic Surgery Today I interviewed Dr. Susan Kolb, who brings a special insight to the subject of implants, since she herself had experience with an implant failure. We discussed the many developments and complications associated with with procedure.

http://webtalkradio.net/internet-talk-radio/2012/03/26/inside-cosmetic-surgery-today-%E2%80%93-breast-implant-problems-%E2%80%93-the-facts-from-dr-lycka-dr-kolb/

I also discussed breast augmentation and reconstruction with Dr. Daryl Hoffman of Palo Alto, who is an authority on the subject. We talked about the advantages of fat grafting as opposed to implants and the limitations of current stem cell technology as applied to breast augmentation.

http://webtalkradio.net/internet-talk-radio/2012/05/07/inside-cosmetic-surgery-today-breast-enhancement-surgery-implant-information-dr-lycka-dr-hoffman/

Fat Grafting and Fat Transfer Augmentation Mammoplasty (FAMI)

ℬecause of the complications associated with breast implants and the reconstruction of breasts following breast cancer surgery and irradiation, many doctors have sought other options. One of these is to harvest fat and in some cases stem cells, and inject them into the breast. This allows the breast to be augmented or reconstructed without the side effects of traditional breast implants. And irradiated breast tissue, which has presented intractable obstacles to reconstruction, is much improved through fat transplant techniques. I recently discussed the implications of this procedure with Dr. Jeffrey Hartog, an expert in this procedure.

http://webtalkradio.net/internet-talk-radio/2012/07/02/inside-cosmetic-surgery-today-fat-grafting-fat-transfer-explained-by-dr-lycka-dr-hartog/

Dr. Hartog's website is http://www.breastreconstruction-andaugmentation.com

Breast reduction Surgery

ℬreast reduction, usually undertaken as a purely medical procedure in cases where overly heavy breasts are a burden for the patient, is done by removing excess breast tissue and skin and reshaping the breast to compensate for the lost tissue. Because of the quantity of tissue that is sometimes removed, recovery is necessarily a little slower.

For years, breast reductions have been a procedure with some of the highest degrees of patient satisfaction. In a well trained cosmetic surgeons hands, it is a great cosmetic procedure. More recently, liposuction has been used alone as a breast reduction technique. In select patients, it has yielded gratifying results.

Breast Lifts and Other Lifting Procedures

*B*reast lifts, termed "mastopexy," does not change the size of the breast or create a rounder upper surface. However, where the nipples of the unsupported breast hang below the bottom crease of the breast, some women choose this procedure to restore a more youthful appearance. In a similar way, redundant tissue can be removed from sagging arms, thighs and legs.

I recently discussed the breast lift as part of a "mommy makeover" with Dr. Ed Miranda of San Francisco. As you'll hear, this has often proved a very gratifying procedure for patients.

http://webtalkradio.net/internet-talk-radio/2012/06/18/inside-cosmetic-surgery-today-mommy-makeover-how-can-it-help-your-post-pregnancy-body-dr-lycka-dr-miranda/

Abdominoplasty and Other Tucks

A tummy tuck (abdominoplasty) removes excess skin from the abdominal area and can tighten weakened or separated muscles to create an abdominal profile that is smoother and firmer. The procedure results in a flatter, smoother stomach. As with liposuction, the purpose of a tummy tuck is to reshape an area of the body rather than to reduce body weight. An abdominoplasty is a significant procedure that entails six to twelve weeks of downtime. An undesirable result can be an outpouching of skin on the corners of an incision, known as "dog ears," unless the surgeon takes special care to prevent them. Abdominoplasties are not insignificant procedures and fortunately laser liposuction and laser techniques have lessened the number of patients requiring this procedure.

Rhinoplasty

Rhinoplasty is in something of a category of its own. The nose is an important feature of the face, being smack dab in the centre, and its repair by plastic surgeons lies near the genesis of modern cosmetic surgery. Rhinoplasty can change the size, shape, and angle of the nose to bring it into better proportion with the rest of the face. It can alter the tip of the nose, correct bumps, indentations or other defects. It's generally assumed that one's nose must be proportional to one's face to be attractive, but different ethnic groups have differently shaped noses and different cultures admire different features. One size certainly doesn't fit all.

Purely medical rhinoplasty may correct structural problems with the nose that may be causing chronic congestion and breathing problems. Surgeons who perform rhinoplasties typically have training in plastic surgery, otorhinolaryngology (the ear, nose, and throat specialty) or both. Recently, a noninvasive rhinoplasty has been used to lift the nose without surgery.

If you're seeking a cosmetic rhinoplasty, and if your expectations are realistic and your plastic surgeon shares them, he or she will probably be able to give you the results you want.

Female Genital Surgery

Dr Susan Kolb and I recently discussed female genital surgery. http://webtalkradio.net/internet-talk-radio/2012/04/16/inside-cosmetic-surgery-today-female-genital-cosmetic-surgery-labiaplasty-dr-lycka-dr-kolb/

Whereas some members of the medical profession have criticized this procedure as mutilation, many patients have requested it for a variety of reasons. Here are some of them:

♦ "I have too much tissue around my clitoris and want to have it removed for better orgasms."

- ◆ "I have too much tissue on my labia and it is uncomfortable when I have sex or play sports."
- ◆ "I don't like the way I look down there."
- ◆ "I stretched out after my baby was delivered."
- ◆ "I took steroids and tissue started to grow down there."
- ◆ "I look funny in a swimsuit."

Sexual Reassignment Surgery

*I*n 2012, Jenna Talackova, 23, was disqualified as a finalist in the 61st Miss Universe Canada pageant because she was born a male. While it is uncertain how much surgery was done to transform her into the beauty she is, it is undeniable that she had some.

I recently discussed transgender surgery with Dr. Jeffrey Spiegel of Yale University. Dr. Spiegel explains that this developing branch of surgical medicine is not focused on the primary sexual organs, as most people might expect, but on the "feminization" of facial features. More subtle characteristics distinguish man and woman than our obvious sexual anatomy.

http://webtalkradio.net/internet-talk-radio/2012/06/04/inside-cosmetic-surgery-today-facial-feminization-surgery-gives-transgender-men-a-feminine-face-dr-lycka-dr-spiegel/

4. I hate the bumpy "cottage cheese" appearance of my buttocks and thighs.

Cellulite Removal

I've given cellulite its own section because in several respects it's a special case. The truth is, we've had little by way

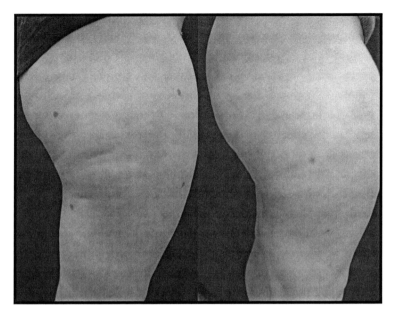

Cellulaze, the recently developed laser technique, may offer a low-risk and effective aprroach to the treatment of cellulite. Here an un-retouched before and after suggests the potential.

effective treatment for the bumpy, orange-peel-like fat that has discouraged and distressed women for so long: cellulite or, less appealingly, "cottage cheese thighs." The effect is produced by normal fat pushing up through the web of connective tissue that formerly kept it distributed beneath the skin. I liken cellulite to an overstuffed mattress or to two pounds of fat in a one pound net bag, the dimpling occurring as the cords pull things down and extra fat rises to make those bumps. Genetics, total body fat and age are all contributive factors but in fact we don't yet understand the precise mechanism responsible for the development of this cosmetic nuisance.

As to treatment for cellulite, good cosmetic practitioners have wisely advised their clients to diet and exercise but, as we've seen from some of our patients' liposuction stories earlier in this book, diet and exercise are often not enough to eliminate stubborn fat.

The same is true of cellulite. Lotions and potions have proved frankly useless. A much-touted medication failed to stand up in clinical trials. Endermologie combined with mesotherapy produces some improvement of cellulite and I myself have offered this combination as the best technology available. Liposuction—even the laser-assisted SmartLipo—although it removes fat, often has the effect of making cellulite worse because the skin remains loose and the "net" of cords remain in place. A difficult surgical procedure called subscision that involves actually cutting the cords has been shown to work but is obviously very difficult to apply over extensive areas.

I've gone into this detail to make my point that, when a cosmetic problem is so complex, the patient's only protection is the doctor's integrity, candor and good will. You can't afford to be paying for procedures that won't work or at least won't work as well as described.

But the cellulite story doesn't necessarily have an unhappy ending. As we know, cosmetic technologies are in a constant state of evolution and in 2011, I sat down with Dr. Bruce Katz of New York City, the man who first introduced me to SmartLipo.

http://webtalkradio.net/internet-talk-radio/2012/08/26/inside-cosmetic-surgery-today-liposuction-reviewed-compared-with-cellulaze-by-dr-lycka-dr-katz/

Bruce described to my listeners the latest advances in Smart-Lipo—changes in light frequency and in the way the laser light is directed from the tip of the optical fiber—that now allow surgeons to remove fat from all levels in one procedure and cut the cords that create the cellulite effect.

Bruce has been among those conducting FDA trials with this new Cellulaze technology. You'll have gathered from some of the comments by other physicians I've interviewed that Cellulaze shows huge promise in eliminating extensive cellulite in a single hour-long session with no complications so far and few after-effects. Best of all, the results of these studies, unpublished as this book goes to press, appear to last at least two years and probably much longer.

This is what we've come to expect of cosmetic medicine: constant improvement by the best and most demanding physicians and researchers.

5. I'm embarrassed by unsightly varicose veins on my legs.

$\mathcal{V}$aricose veins are not in themselves a disease, but rather a symptom of a disease called "superficial venous insufficiency of lower extremities." The muscles of the legs return blood to the heart against the force of gravity and tiny valves—"leaflets"—prevent backflow of the blood. Only about ten percent of blood return is handled by the superficial veins that are near the surface, and it is these veins that are most subject to high pressure when standing and most likely to experience failure of the leaflets and thus superficial venous insufficiency. The blood backs up and the

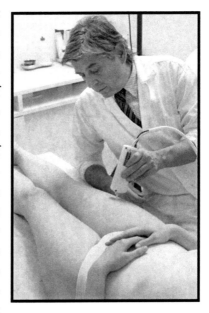

A practitioner diagnoses varicosity in a patient's leg as the first step of the EVLT procedure.

result is the swollen, torturous appearance of varicosity. Varicose veins can be a significant cause of pain and discomfort in legs. According to Dr. Chao Yu, an expert in vein therapy, patients complain of aching, fatigue, cramps and swelling of the legs and are often in search of symptomatic relief. The other issue, of course, is aesthetic improvement. ("I have this ugly patch I would like to improve.")

The standard treatment was surgically stripping out the affected veins (ligation), a potentially painful procedure with some risk. Today, other techniques have largely replaced stripping.

Sclerotherapy

Sclerotherapy is a procedure for the treatment of small varicose veins and spider veins, which are closely related. A chemical is injected into a vein to damage and scar the interior lining of the vein, which causes it to close. The blood is returned by the larger, interior veins. As a procedure, sclerotherapy is far less likely to produce complications.

If you're considering, sclerotherapy, your number one question should be, Is this the doctor's specialty?

Endovenous Laser Therapy (EVLT)

Here we meet again our friends the lasers, even more satisfactory in many cases of varicosity than sclerotherapy. The word "laser" is an acronym for "light amplification by stimulated emission of radiation." Through a chemical process, a beam of light of a single wavelength is produced and can be aimed and tuned to affect a specific target and not others. Lasers selectively treat blood vessels by using specific wavelengths of red and sometimes blue light. The EVLT procedure uses a minimally invasive "endovenous"—literally "within the vein"—laser and is a clinically proven alternative. It requires no general anesthesia and offers minimal risk and shorter recovery time. The EVLT procedure uses the latest generation of EVLT catheter, a laser fiber inserted directly into the faulty vein under local anesthesia. The laser delivers a precise dose of energy into the vein wall, collapsing it. This process, called ablation, cures the condition and diverts blood flow to nearby functional veins. The resulting increased circulation significantly reduces the symptoms of varicose veins and improves their surface appearance.

EVLT combines a number of skills and I am grateful to Dr. Chao Yu, whose vascular surgery practice is in Edmonton, for offering me the benefit of his experience. The most challenging part of EVLT for the surgeon is the first step, canulizing the vein. The second step, injecting the tumuscent anaesthetic, requires ultrasound skill as a visual aid. Unless your surgeon is a radiologist,he or she will need to hire an ultrasonographer. As with so many cosmetic procedures, the more experienced a practitioner is, the better the results are likely to be. Expect to pay somewhere between $2000 and $4000.

6. I have excessive and unwanted hair on my face or body.

There are a few medical issues with excessive hair, but once they are ruled out, this is truly one of mankind's oldest and largest cosmetic complaints. Men have been shaving hair from their faces in various cultures and during various periods for thousands of years. The record as it pertains to women is less complete—not surprising since, except for their heads, women generally have far less, and less obvious, hair.

There are four popular approaches to lessening or removing unwanted hair: shaving, chemical depilatories, electrolysis, and lasers. I deal with these hair issues at some length in my book, SkinWorks. Shaving and depilatories are established tools that may be used at home with a number of caveats and cautions. Here are the other two, which you might encounter in a medical context:

Electrolysis

Electrolysis (the actual mechanism, the practice is properly called "electrology") remains popular and is highly effective and permanent as a method of hair removal. It may employ electricity ("galvanic electrolysis") or microwave energy ("thermolysis") or a mix of the two, administered through a hair-fine probe inserted in the follicle. Over a period of several years, the electrolysis process can permanently remove hair. Numerous clinics offer one of the several electrolysis techniques and I would advise you to apply to any of them the general interrogation I recommend for all cosmetic practices on pages 166–171.

Laser Hair Removal

Lasers are becoming the approach of choice because they are easier, less painful, and less tedious than electrolysis, though the results may be less complete and less permanent. The cautions I offer to those looking for a laser hair treatment are those I apply generally to laser procedures (see page _, above).

I personally began to do laser hair removal in the early 1990s. The lasers were primitive compared to those of today and in order to work, a dark carbon had to be applied to the skin. Now we have learned to target the hairs while preserving the skin with dynamic cooling equipment. The result: better results, less complications. Nonetheless, laser hair removal is not complication free. As always, the buyer must be aware.

7. I'm losing my hair!

That's people for you, isn't it? If we're not trying to get rid of hair, we're trying to grow it. Of course, the hair that nature is most inclined to get rid of forever is the very hair we'd like to keep: our top locks.

> "I was so angry! I was only twenty and already
> I was losing my hair. I really didn't want to

look like my father at such an early age."

"For a long time I denied that I was losing my hair. I knew my mother's hair was pretty thin but I really didn't think it would happen to me."

"When my hairstylist told me I was losing my hair, I ate a tub of ice cream. Losing my hair? Not me, please!"

"I'm a very proud person. I really try to do my best and look my best. So when I noticed a lot more in my brush and in my tub, I just lost it. Why was this happening to me. It was so unfair!"

Hair loss may be due to causes other than the purely genetic—*androgenetic alopecia*, as inherited male pattern baldness is technically called when it happens to men. Metabolic, autoimmune or infectious causes are all possible. Thyroid disease, hormonal imbalances, alopecia areata (an autoimmune disease), scalp infections, skin diseases, medications (for cancer, arthritis, high blood pressure, depression and heart problems), physical or mental shock, certain hair styles and emotional issues: any of them can cause hair loss. It's clearly important to seek expert medical opinion before embarking on a course of treatment. But bear in mind that hair restoration products have been flogged to the vulnerable public since time immemorial, so curb your expectations and proceed with caution.

Finasteride and minoxidil

These medications are FDA approved for the stabilization of hair loss or restoration of lost hair in cases of common-or-garden-variety, genetically determined, male-pattern baldness. Sold under numerous trade names including Rogaine/Regaine, Vanarex,

Mintop, Loniten, Proscar and Propecia, they are generally more effective when hair loss is not too advanced. Their effects wear off within months of stopping use of the medication. Anyone considering using these products should seek medical advice and follow-up. A review of the possible adverse side effects is sobering.

Low Laser Light Therapy (LLLT)

We encountered LLLT back in our discussion about treating aging and damaged skin. But based on a number of small studies and one good double-blind study in 2009, evidence has emerged that low-energy laser light in the red part of the spectrum can help stimulate hair growth in men and women with pattern baldness. The mechanism is not yet fully understood but there is some evidence that the laser light reverses the programmed cell death of the hair follicles. There are hand-held laser devices for home use and the therapy is also available in medical settings. In either case, results are achieved through multiple sessions over months and sustained through maintenance use. Physicians may also use LLLT in conjunction with hair transplantation.

Surgical Hair Transplants

Hair transplantation is the apex of hair loss therapy. In expert hands, it can be a one-time fix that lasts for many years and only be evident later if more hair is lost from the adjacent untransplanted areas. The techniques have evolved continuously, like so many others in cosmetic medicine, and today's ultra-refined follicular unit hair transplantation (follicular units are the tiny natural groupings on hair follicles), with over fifty grafts per square centimeter, is the present gold standard. There is very little discomfort or downtime.

It goes without saying that hair transplantation is an advanced surgical technique that is best performed by highly trained and skilled surgeons. Hair loss treatment in general is highly specialized and it's worth your time to search out the best. You want a doctor who shares information, communicates readily and has a history of getting results. You want a doctor who can acknowledge that these can be difficult procedures but can demonstrate that his or her team have perfected the ones they use. You want a doctor who has done hundreds to thousands of cases. You want a doctor, as always, who can manage your expectations.

8. I thought tattoos were cool but I've changed my mind.

Tattoo Removal

We see a lot of tattoos these days and you sometimes wonder that something so permanent is so fashion-based and impulsive in origin. Fortunately, in these days of the laser, tattoos can usually be completely or almost completely erased with four to thirty sessions of treatment using a high energy Nd/YAG, Alexandrite or ruby laser over several weeks or months. There are sometimes residual pigmentation effects. I've described elsewhere how I did this for years on a *pro bono* basis to help poor former prostitutes and gang members escape a past they no longer wanted. There are many lasers that can remove tattoos but no one system can remove all tattoos. Recently, multiple lasers are being sold to doctors in one box to help them obtain optimal results.

9. An accident or surgery has left me with scars that won't go away.

I see patients who hate their scars.
"I was so ashamed. I had horrific acne when I was a kid. It left my face horribly scarred. I know people thought I was from another planet by the way they looked at me."

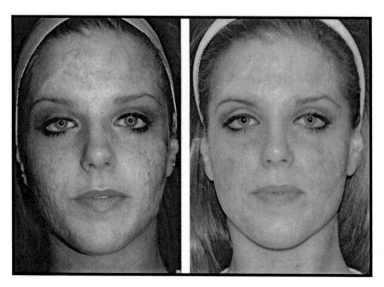

Modern cosmetic dermatology has permitted the remarkable amelioration of traumatic scar damage. Courtesy Dr. Jill Waibel.

> "When I was in the car accident, I was thrown through the windshield. My forehead literally exploded and I needed 114 sutures to close it. I guess I was lucky but every time I look in the mirror I see these horrendous scars."

> "When I was a kid, I did a very foolish thing and slashed my wrist. I still get depressed when I look at them."

Whether scars have come about as a result of an accident or cystic acne or some other cause, they can inflict psychological stress. Patients may feel everyone stares at them when they enter a room. They may blame the scars for their failure to find a job or meet a mate. They may believe the scars simply make them look ugly.

Scar Treatment

*T*reating unsightly scars is an important part of cosmetic practice that was once the sole province of the plastic surgeon. Scars may be red with lots of blood vessels), coloured (meaning they contain greater numbers of pigment cells than surrounding tissues, elevated or keloidal as a result of too much scar tissue, or depressed below surrounding tissue. Cosmetic doctors who treat scars must know how to target all these elements. The scope of this book doesn't allow me to detail the many techniques and procedures that can be employed, except to say that fillers, grafting, resurfacing, laser, radiation, steroid injections, Botox injections and surgery all have a place. A doctor approaches a scar with one end result in mind: cosmetic improvement. To get there he takes the component of the scar firmly in hand: the colour, the scar type, the elevation, the texture. Then he uses all the tools in his saddle bag to address them. Since there isn't a single approach, I can't provide you with a single set of guidelines, except to say that like all the procedures in this book, results will vary. And the biggest and most important variable is your choice of a cosmetic doctor.

I recommend you ask the doctor if this will be one treatment or a series of treatments. Ask what the chances are that these treatments will be successful. Don't be afraid to ask how many scar corrections of this type the doctor has done and whether you can talk to someone who has had the procedure.

10.   I have a harmless mole or skin tag that I nonetheless find unsightly.

Mole Removal

*T*he removal of benign skin lesions—lumps and bumps more properly called seborrheic keratoses, benign intradermal nevi, skin tags, sebaceous hyperplasia, dermatosa papulosa nigra and others—is the most common cosmetic procedure of them all. The techniques vary from liquid nitrogen to laser to actual surgery and cost is relatively low, but as a patient you must bear two points in mind:

Probably less that ten percent of moles are malignant but even your G.P. may not always be able to reliably distinguish harmless from harmful. Given that one type of malignant mole is the deadly skin cancer, melanoma, take your concerns to your dermatologist. In *SkinWorks*, I discuss how to recognize skin lesions that should arouse your suspicions.

Second, the removal of moles without leaving an unsightly scar is expert work. Sometimes it's almost impossible. That's why it's so important to find a surgeon who's concerned first and foremost about you, not just ready to do whatever you want if you pay the fee. Ask how he or she plans to do the removal. Ask about the risks. Ask if your doctor can guarantee no scar. Trick question: no one can.

Last Thoughts

*I*f you don't have a concern in one of these ten areas we've discussed, I'll be surprised. There are of course other and numerous sub-divisions of the ones I've listed. But again, I hope my message is clear: cosmetic medicine is rapidly evolving—a moving target, if you like—and only your efforts can be expected to produce the solution that suits you best.

There are numerous cosmetic surgery techniques, technologies, substances, procedures, medications and conditions that I haven't space to treat with in this book. Those I have discussed have been by way of illustration: the questions and cautions you use in choosing whom you would trust to do one of these will also apply to anything else in the field.

At this point in the book, we've canvassed enough opinions

and set out as many rules and words of advice as you'll want to read. Now it's time for you to act. Step out the front door and step in the door of two or three cosmetic practices and, armed with your Doctor Index, ask some pointed questions.

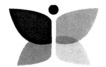

6 THE DOCTOR INDEX

𝒯he most important determinant of cosmetic surgery success is the choice of the doctor who will do your cosmetic surgery. In your search for the ideal cosmetic practitioner, I like to say there are two cardinal rules

♦ Consider more than one candidate.

♦ Go in asking questions.

But how to compare candidates when you yourself may not have medical expertise? My sense is that you're likely to be guided in your final decision by gut instinct: some combination of your own personality and the impressions you receive from a particular doctor, staff and clinic. Nonetheless, I want to bring a more analytical tool to your side by summing up what we've learned in the book. The result is the Doctor Index, a simple inventory that allows you to quantify and compare your assessment of more than one doctor.

As preparation for creating your own personal version of the Doctor Index, I'd like to review some of the things I've learned—and hopefully have passed on to you in the course of this book—about how anyone should approach the choice of a cosmetic doctor. I call these points the Six Secrets of Cosmetic Surgery Success

Secret #1: Your doctor's qualifications count.

𝒥t goes without saying your doctor should be skilled in the procedures he offers. He should have done hundreds of cases and be an authority in the area in question. He should have written on the topic and have shared his techniques with his colleagues. He should teach others about the surgery. It also goes without saying that he should be a member of several professional organizations and ideally serve on their committees.

Secret #2: Your doctor's qualifications don't stop with a diploma.

Knowing if your doctor is a family doctor, a plastic surgeon or a dermatologist is a key piece of information. It may even surprise you to learn that most cosmetic procedures are not taught in residency or medical school, which anyway just gives new doctors the basis on which to build new knowledge. As we saw in my conversations with some of the best, most procedures are too new and cosmetic science keeps progressing. The half life of medical knowledge may be three to five years or less. This means that every few years half the medical knowledge is replaced with new knowledge.

Even if cosmetic procedures were taught in school, that wouldn't mean that your doctor had become an expert in the area., since most of your doctor's education is outside of residency. Remember how in 1986, after watching a liposuction procedure, I vowed never to do liposuction? Why would I do something that would risk a patient's life simply to make them look better? But when Jeffrey Klein developed a means to do liposuction entirely under local anesthesia, I took every course I could, studying under Jeffrey Klein, Bill Coleman III, Patrick Lillis, and Bill Hanke. Only then did I start to do liposuction myself and my education didn't end there. I continued to study with the masters. I learned from Dr. Fournier in Paris and many others. When extrinsic ultrasound became available, I added it to my repertoire. When powered instruments came along, I studied those as well and added them too. Then when lipo-lasers became the state of the art, I studied them and added them. This is what I mean by medical education *after* school.

Secret #3: What others say counts.

A doctor's skill should be manifest in the glowing testimonials from his patients. A doctor who releases such testimonials isn't bragging: he or she is telling you that others like yourself have trod this path and were happy about it.

> "His treatment of laser lipo can do what diet, exercise, and life style change can't. I should know—I'm a physical education teacher. [My problem with excess fat] was not due to a lack of trying! Some areas just need a little help and that help is my doctor and his staff."
>
> T. K., age 41
> May, 2009

> "Very professional and caring! I got what they promised me. After getting rid of all that ugly fat, I feel like a new man!"
>
> M. N., age 25
> June, 2009

> "My tummy is definitely smaller and I believe will get smaller yet, since it still feels a little swollen. I'm thinking of getting more procedures, and would definitely return to my doctor."
>
> K. L., age 52
> June, 2009

> "The result is perfect. It's just the way I always wanted it. My doctor knows and gives advice on what is best for you. Thank you to my doctor and his staff!"
>
> L. D., age 35
> July, 2009

> "With Smart Lipo, the healing was so fast! I was afraid of the results based on the old lipo procedure—but this was a great choice."
>
> H. O., age 53
> July, 2009

"I was very welcomed and never felt any pressure to have the surgery. I feel proud of my new look and would do it again in a heartbeat."

L. C., age 42

July, 2010

"My face seems much more youthful and people have said I look

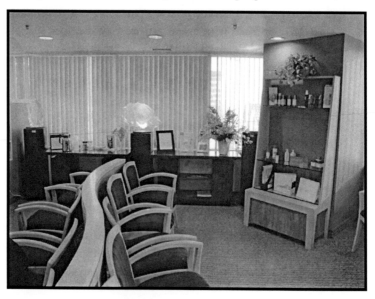

I think the reception area of my own practice in Edmonton leaves little doubt that you're entering the offices of a fully dedicated cosmetic doctor.

more relaxed and very young for my age. With the laser liposuction my clothes fit and hang so much better than before. I look great in my bathing suit (so my husband says!). I sincerely thank my doctor and his wonderful staff for their care and attention to my needs.

Corinne, age 50

September, 2009

"My doctor is very knowledgeable and skilled with the lipo procedure I had done on my flanks and thighs. I am thrilled with the results and feel more confident about my body image. It also feels incredibly comfortable having the excess fat removed from this problem area."

V. M.

September, 2009

"Great service and polite staff! They make you feel very comfortable about having cosmetic procedures done. No need to feel embarrassed about it."

M. J.

October, 2009

"My doctor is one of the top dermatologists in Edmonton. All his staff are very professional and extremely helpful. I even appreciated when one of the nurses phoned the day after my lipo procedure. Great job!"

P. H.

October, 2009

"Very happy with the outcome. My mid-section is flatter and firmer. After a lot of research and a consultation with my doctor I decided on a procedure called LipoDissolve. I could start to see a difference after two treatments and was very happy with the end results. Thanks so much!"

K. K.

November, 2009

"I am very happy that I was able to come and fix my tummy area after having children. With my having had two C-sections, this area was damaged and I had been very embarrassed of my body ever since. My doctor has offered a healthy alternative without major surgery to improve not only my physical appearance but emotional well being. I now feel better wearing my clothes and especially in a bathing suit!"

(anon.)

January, 2010

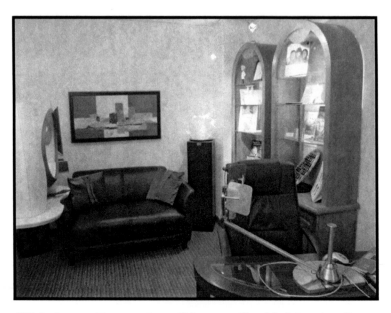

This is the consulting room in my Edmonton office. It's designed to allow my patients to feel at ease. Would it work for you?

"Best money I every spent! I used to walk around with my head held down and now I feel I can raise my head with pride! I feel like my doctor really cares about people and cares about making them feel good about themselves."

(anon.)

February, 2010

"It is the best thing I have done for myself in my life. It has improved my confidence and posture. I'm no longer trying to hide my belly! I don't have to hold everything in and can now buy clothes that fit."

(anon.)

February, 2010

These people are trying to tell us something.

Secret #4: How an office treats you before surgery is an important indication of your procedure's outcome.

This at a first glance may surprise you, but your doctor's personality permeates all aspects of his or her office. The standards set for the staff are the standards that will be reflected in the ongoing relationship with you.

I've always considered my desk staff to be "directors of first impressions." I heard this term used first by Michael McClean, a brilliant mentor to the independent insurance industry. I've always considered the best front desk staff member to be one who can reach over the phone and literally touch the person on the other side. Yes, they are to make a impression and facilitate booking the appointment, but more importantly, they're there to help you.

The other office staff must also be efficient and friendly and help wherever and whenever they can. The nurses must suggest the milk of human kindness. They must be your advocate and helper.

A doctor's office represents that doctor's values and beliefs. A doctor's staff represents her or him. That's why it's so important to observe that office.

Secret #5: The appearance of the doctor's office can give you important clues.

- ♦ A visit to your doctor's office is essential. When you're there, look around.
- ♦ Is there a bouquet of fresh flowers in the reception area?
- ♦ Is there a bulletin board telling you things of interest to you?
- ♦ Are there works of art that suggest the doctor's appreciation of aesthetics?
- ♦ Are there photos of celebs and winning teams? Articles written about your doctor in the press?
- ♦ Is there a video display of the procedures the doctor offers?
- ♦ Is there something to nourish you available?

♦ Are there pamphlets that provide information about cosmetic procedures?

♦ Is there a welcoming front-desk person?

Secret #6: A happy and enthusiastic staff suggests a happy outcome for you.

$\mathcal{H}$enry Ford said this about enthusiasm:

> Enthusiasm is the yeast that makes your hopes rise to the stars. Enthusiasm is the sparkle in your eyes, the swing in your gait, the grip of your hand, the irresistible surge of will and energy to execute your ideas. Enthusiasts are fighters. They have fortitude. They have staying qualities. Enthusiasm is at the bottom of all progress. With it, there is accomplishment. Without it, there are only alibis.

$\mathcal{C}$asey Stengel said: "Finding good players is easy. Getting them to play as a team is another story." And that team's only role should be is to serve you, the patient.

The Questions

$\mathcal{W}$e've established that your choice of doctor is your number one determinant of cosmetic surgery success. Your doctor will interview you to see if you are a reasonable candidate for surgery and I'm a big advocate of you interviewing your doctor to see if he or she is a reasonable candidate to perform the surgery or treatment. Even if you had all the answers, asking your doctor questions would still be of value: how he or she answers will give you a better feel for the person you might be trusting your health and safety to.

1.   How long have you been doing this procedure and what training do you have?

$\mathcal{A}$s I suggested when passing on some secrets to the success of cosmetic procedures, that just because a doctor is a Fellow of the

Royal College of Physicians of Canada (FRCPC), a Diplomat of the American Board of Dermatology, or a member of the American Society of Plastic Surgeons does not necessarily mean he or she is trained in, say, laser surgery or liposuction. Much of the training doctors receive takes place after they complete a fellowship and indeed, little training is available in many popular cosmetic procedures. Recently I had a new graduate join our office. He had perfect marks in medical school and university and had passed his fellowship exams with flying colours but had had no training in lasers or cosmetic procedures. This is typical, even of the best.

When prospective patients ask me where and when I trained, I gladly share all the details. I expect the same of others.

2a. How do you safeguard against complications?

Nothing strikes fear in the heart of a doctor more than complications. However, a good doctor does not take complications lightly. If a doctor tells you, "Complications don't happen in my hands," I strongly suggest you continue your search.

The proper approach for doctors is to guard against complications by meticulous attention to detail. I don't drink alcohol. I go to bed early so I'm well rested. I approach each case with great care, as though I were operating on a trusted friend.

Still, complications happen in the best of hands, mine included. So a follow up to this question is:

2b. What do you do if they do occur?

Serious complications, such as heart attack, pulmonary emboli or death have never occurred in any of my cases. Infections have been so rare as to have been almost non-existent. Minor complications, such as irregularities in the cosmetic result, occur in about 5% of patients.

If a major complication were to occur, I would use all the skills my advance cardiac life support (ACLS) training has provided. If a minor irregularity occurs following a liposuction procedure, we would deal with it by using lipodissolve or by redoing the liposuction procedure. If there should be some other minor complication, we would discuss treatment carefully. I'm in your corner working for you until we get it right and I expect your doctor to do the same.

3.   How will I be followed after my procedure?

This is a very important question, because the procedure does not end with the treatment or surgery. Your body must adjust to the surgery that has been done and every case is different.

As I tell my patients, what I do is fairly predictable. What the body does with what I do is not. So, after a procedure, we watch and wait. I always give printed instructions on what a person is to do after surgery and have my office call them the next day. I encourage my patients to call me if they have any problems and we give every person a 24-hour phone number where they can reach me.

Depending on the type of surgery done, we arrange a follow-up appointment or series of follow-up appointments at mutually convenient times. We assess progress at each appointment, and are forever mindful of possible intervening complications.

My office staff are instructed to treat every surgery patient as a VIP. If a patient is concerned about anything, we call them in to see me. It doesn't matter how busy I am; these patients require special care and treatment.

Ask your doctor if he or she plans to do the same. I'm afraid you may be surprised by many answers.

4. What does your doctor do for the community?

If you hadn't read this book, this would have seemed like a peculiar question. But a doctor who is truly aware is not only concerned about you, but concerned about the larger community. Remember the 2000 movie *Pay It Forward*, in which a twelve-year-old boy undertakes a challenge from his teacher to do something that will change the world? All doctors need to feel like they're in that movie.

As I mentioned in my conversation with Sarah Burge, I myself give free cosmetic surgery to women who are victims of domestic abuse and free tattoo removal to prostitutes who want to free themselves from bondage to the streets. I am an avid supporter of the arts and was a major financial supporter during the push to bring *The Lion King* to Edmonton. I support the YWCA Women of Distinction Program and formed the Canadian Skin Cancer Foundation to support programs to eliminate skin cancer. (One example of this is our $70,000 gift to support the Cross Cancer Institute's Chair in Dermatology for Melanoma Research). Also, I take time to mentor the younger generation of cosmetic surgeons through MasterMind clubs.

You'll recall my conversations with Jeff Riopelle, who "bought" Halloween candy back from children in his practice and from the children of his patients. With a service organization, he sent the candy to the troops in Afghanistan and the money he gave for the candy actually went to the school the child attended.

One of my former MasterMind students is Dr. Peter Ursel from Lindsay, Ontario. Peter runs in office events and charges admission for people to attend. He then gives this money to charity. I do something similar. A recent seminar raised $7000 for tsunami relief.

Whatever the avenue they choose, ask your doctor how he's involved in the larger community and his reasons for doing so.

5. What happens if I'm not happy after my procedure?

No doctor likes to think something can or will go wrong. I certainly don't, but I'm well aware that it remains a possibility. And although a setback happens rarely, I will work with any unhappy client until they are satisfied. I've found that we can overcome most disappointments with time and effort. You'll want to know whether your doctor shares this attitude.

6. What testimonials do you have from other patients?

I know this seems like a brutal question, but consider this: If patients are happy with the results of a doctor's work, many of them will be willing to say so. Cosmetic doctors want to reassure prospective patients and have every reason to collect such testimonials. Does your doctor have lots of them to show? Good—that's as it should be. No? Why not?

Compiling Your Index

I'm going to assume now that you haven't just trotted along to the office with the lowest advertised price or biggest ads, but have instead interviewed a few doctors about the procedure or problem you're interested in. You've carried your little crib sheet with questions drawn from this book and you've made a note of the answers.

Now, as I've said, I'm realistic. I know you're going to be swayed in part by many factors, not all of them wholly rational. We're all a bit like that. But just to add some simple quantification to the mix, take some time to create your Doctor Index. If nothing else, it will help confirm your decision made on gut instinct and perhaps serve as a reminder that the choice of a cosmetic practitioner should be based on a careful inquiry, not a television ad.

To make it easier to handle, the Index is arranged in five categories: reputation, communication, curiosity, knowledge & competence, sharing & caring, and the pursuit of excellence: categories based on my observations as a physician and on my discussions with other physicians—and with patients. You'll note that the factors often cross-link with one another: communication skills may be closely related to sharing and caring, for example.

But score them separately anyway. It's always possible that a caring doctor could be a poor communicator.

As you compile your Index, you'll see that some items award more than a single point. It's up to you to decide whether a full score is merited or not. Adjust your scoring accordingly.

So you've sharpened your questions—now sharpen your pencil. Here we go.

1. THE REPUTATION FACTOR Before you even see the doctor	Score	Doctor 1	Doctor 2
Word of mouth; you heard about this doctor from an acquaintance whose opinion you take seriously. The opinion could be positive or negative.	-1 to +1		
You were referred to this doctor by a medical professional.	2		
You saw this doctor cited in independent media (TV, radio, print) or saw this doctor's writing independently published.	2		
You saw this doctor listed positively or negatively on an Internet "doctor rating" site.	0		
You saw this doctor's ad in the phone book, on TV or radio, or on the Internet.	0		
While visiting the doctor, you saw abundant evidence of testimonials from former patients.	3		
Saw this doctor on a radio or television interview.	3		
MAXIMUM 11			

2. THE COMMUNICATION FACTOR You can't decide if you don't know enough			
	Score	Doctor 1	Doctor 2
You had a direct interview with the doctor.	3		
The doctor used the interview to describe options and to explain any particular procedure in as much detail as necessary for you.	3		
The doctor described possible side-effects of the procedure and how these are dealt with in writing or in person.	3		
The doctor's web site(s) contained features that were clearly designed to educate patients, not just sell them on procedures.	2		
The doctor's office offered educational materi-al—videos, brochures, books, websites, radio and televiion interviews, etc.—that went beyond sales tools.	4		
The doctor's staff provided additional information related to your procedure.	2		
POSSIBLE MAXIMUM 17			

3. THE CURIOSITY FACTOR			
The itch that every good cosmetic surgeon must satisfy.			
	Score	Doctor 1	Doctor 2
The doctor proves that he attends on-going training and seminars.	2		
When asked, he or she is able to name a specific program attended in the previous year.	2		
The doctor is a member of a MasterMind club with other cosmetic surgeons.	6		
The doctor, when asked, is able to speak of techniques and/or equipment investigated and rejected/accepted.	2		
The doctor has adopted a new procedure in the last 3 years.	3		
POSSIBLE MAXIMUM 15			

4. THE KNOWLEDGE & COMPETENCE FACTOR			
In a constantly advancing field, the doctor learns by doin.			
	Score	Doctor 1	Doctor 2
How long has the doctor had a cosmetic practice—not general surgery or plastic surgery? Score 4 points for every ten years up to 20 years.	0 to 8		
How long has the doctor been doing this procedure? Score 1 point for every 2 years up to 20 years.	0 to 10		
On how many patients has the doctor performed this procedure? Score 2 points for every 40 patients up to 200 patients.	0 to 10		
The doctor has published or presented on this procedure in a peer-reviewed journal.	3		
POSSIBLE MAXIMUM 31			

5. THE SHARING & CARING FACTOR				
Your health and well-being must come before a doctor's bank account				
		Score	Doctor 1	Doctor 2
The doctor does regular community and charity work.		3		
The doctor performs cosmetic procedures on a pro bono basis for special cases.		3		
The doctor holds or has recently held teaching positions related to his profession.		2		
The doctor mentors other doctors as they learn cosmetic techniques.		3		
The doctor's personal interview with you demonstrates careful attention to your points.		2		
The doctor's staff demonstrates a caring and concerned attitude.		4		
POSSIBLE MAXIMUM 17				

6. THE EXCELLENCE FACTOR
The pursuit of perfection is at the heart of the profession.

	Score	Doctor 1	Doctor 2
Thoroughness: the doctor or staff are concerned to understand and record your medical history and overall health.	3		
The doctor is prepared to advise you against procedures he/she believes to be unsuitable for you.	3		
The doctor states that he/she is there to do whatever you want.	(-3)		
The doctor's reception areas and offices demonstrate a clear concern for good taste and agreeable surroundings.	2		
The doctor will be available for follow-up on your procedure, being neither too busy nor too far away.	4		
The doctor's policy is to work with patients post-procedure to adjust results as necessary.	4		
This doctor's services are provided through a large clinic with prominent advertising.	0		
POSSIBLE MAXIMUM 16			

Doctor Index Totals All Factors	Maximum Possible	Doctor 1	Doctor 2
	100		

That's it, then. Judges, total your scores!

So, one doctor scored 73 and one scored 81? Okay, now comes the real calculation. How do you feel about the scores you actually got? Do they confirm your hunch? Or do you say, "Hm, he got ten points lower, but you know what? I sort of like him better."

That's your man. The Index is here to help you, not rule your better judgement. It's the process that counts.

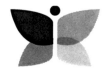

7 BEFORE WE GO

The Trends

No book addressing cosmetic surgery can adequately discuss procedures without at least some discussion of cosmetic surgery trends. Every year I cover these on my web site, YourCosmeticDoctor.tv.

On my weekly radio show *Inside Cosmetic Surgery Today* on WebTalkRadio.net, (http://webtalkradio.net/internet-talk-radio/inside-cosmetic-surgery-today/). I interview guests whose views on this topic are relevant to my listeners. These perspectives are important because, as techniques and procedures change and evolve, innovations may be appropriate for some cosmetic patients, while others,

informed about the current state of the art, may want to wait until the procedures have evolved further. I recently reviewed some of the latest trends on the show and, based on that broadcast, here follows an assortment of cosmetic trends that are attracting attention right now—and a few predictions about where it's headed.

1. Less Will Be Even More

In 2013, one of the major trends in cosmetic thinking will continue to be "less is more." The "overdone" look will be increasingly viewed as less desirable, while the more "natural" look will stay on the rise. A footnote though: Dr. Daryl Hoffman of Palo Alto,

California, whom I interviewed earlier, believes this to be true of the face but not the breast. "In this respect, women still love to be endowed," says Dr. Hoffman.

But in France, where smaller breasts have become increasingly popular, the "less is more" philosophy is alive and well.

2. *The Invasion of the Minimally Invasive*

Botox is the prime example of the minimally invasive procedure and Botox use is up 12 per cent. Dysport is a related product and both are safe and successful. And a new weapon in the neuro-modulator anti-wrinkle locker is Xeomin, which blocks the signals from nerves to the muscles that cause vertical frown lines. That's right, it freezes wrinkles out!

I myself have backed the minimalist innovations heavily, including the new Ulthera and Cellulaze techniques. Cellulaze, as you may have noticed in my doctor interviews, is all the rage and the results make me eager to continue to explore their application.

3. *The Men Strike Back*

I predict more men than ever will be undergoing cosmetic procedures, but I don't have to stick my neck out to say that. No less than the American Association of Plastic Surgeons is saying the same thing. What procedures are men turning to? Facelifts, liposuction, Botox and breast reduction. We baby boomers are famous for our yearning to perpetuate our youth and I believe there'd already be more men seeking procedures if it were not for fear of pain. Come on, guys. We're boomers but we're not babies.

4. *It's All About Skin*

I predict a continuing surge in amazing products to apply to the skin. Pro-Niacin is a revolutionary molecule that penetrates deeply to repair UV-induced DNA damage associated with skin cancer.

The pigment in our skin is protective, but too much pigment

as the result of sun damage, for instance, is unsightly. New herbal formulations have been shown to be effective and produce far less inflammatory side-effects than prescription products.

People experiencing inflammation after laser resurfacing can use a new barrier cream that enhances healing and restores the skin's natural defences.

5. *The New Will Get Newer*

I predict that some of the cutting-edge products now appearing will prove more popular in the long run than fillers or face lifts. Selphyl, for example, is a technique that restores volume to the face, not with synthetics, but by injecting you with your own harvested plasma, which contains growth hormones. In a similar way, a patient's own stem cells can be used to repair damage beneath the dermis that causes wrinkles and volume depletion.

6. *They Won't Be Able to Keep a Good Filler Down*

But I predict fillers will remain popular, with a new generation of products that I'm excited about. Over a thousand based on hyaluronic acid are now available in Europe. In a clinical study of Voluma filler, physicians rated an astonishing 89 per cent of patients much improved or very much improved after treatment.

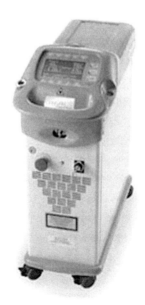

7. *The Advance of the Laser*

I predict the professional interest in lasers will continue to grow. Yes, my evidence is anecdotal but many doctors I chat with are now buying the latest generations of lasers—and

Another Smart Lipo machine

no wonder! I myself use these incredibly versatile tools for skin resurfacing, eyelid surgery, removal of unwanted blood vessels, smart liposuction and tattoo removal.

8. Open Wide for Beauty

I foretell that cosmetic treatments will be increasingly available at—your dentist! Botox is already used for some dental disorders and now some dentists are going a step further and using it for aesthetic purposes. Some are venturing into fillers too. Do I mind? Not at all. Dentists know facial anatomy and about giving injections. *That* can't be said about providers who go into homes and motels, sometimes with disfiguring results.

9. No Sweat About the Future

I predict that human beings will continue to sweat and that hyperhydrosis—that's the term for excessive perspiration—will continue to embarrass. That's why I believe Ulthera, a minimally invasive procedure that uses ultrasound energy to kill off problem sweat glands from the inside, will be increasingly popular. You may have heard of Ulthera being used to lift the skin, but this versatile equipment will be shown to have multiple uses. Will the effects be a permanent answer to hyperhydrosis? Ah, that I won't predict.

10. The Folly of Youth

A recent survey suggests that 90% of ten to eighteen-year-old girls are unhappy with how they look. Air-brushed images are said to be giving them an unrealistic ideal of female beauty. I predict this will lead to publicity about premature cosmetic surgery. Do I approve of such surgery? No.

11. Downtime Down

*D*owntime will go down too because people are also worried about *keeping* jobs. Consumers will demand ever keener prices (but be wary: too cheap means poor quality) and as little down-time as possible—or none at all.

12. *Cosmetic Procedures Up*

Times may be tough but there's been a five percent rise in cosmetic surgery procedures over the last year. The explanation may be a simple one: people want jobs and looking youthful is a competitive advantage. Meanwhile, Oscar-winning actresses and pop icons are one-upping their rivals by coming out against cosmetic procedures. They are, of course, already rich and famous. Despite their sniffing, I fearlessly predict the number of ordinary people opting for cosmetic procedures will continue to increase. Am I taking a risk with that one? I don't think so.

In Conclusion

Thank you for coming along with me on this little journey of discovery and preparation. I'll leave you now with the hope and wish that your adventure in cosmetic medicine is a joyful and rewarding one. If you would like further guidance from me, I invite you to visit my website at www.barrylyckamd.com or consult the other doctors who've participated in this discussion.

And in closing, I don't think I could do better than to repeat the thought expressed by Dr. Steve Schlosser: All your information and questions, with the responses you've received, add up to one thing: your trust. Would you trust this person to look after you? Do you believe he or she cares? If the answer is yes, you've found your doctor.

GLOSSARY

$\mathcal{M}$ost of the terms I introduce in this book are explained as we go. Here however are some thumbnail definitions for others mentioned in passing.

Antioxidant: a molecule that inhibits the oxidation of other molecules. Oxidation reactions can produce free radicals molecules that can start chain reactions in a cell and so cause damage or death to the cell.

Cosmeceuticals: coined term for cosmetics that possess some of the therapeutic qualities of pharmaceuticals.

Cytokines: small cell-signaling protein molecules that are secreted by numerous cells and comprise a category of signaling molecule used extensively in intercellular communication.

Collagen: a group of naturally occurring proteins and the main component of the body's connective tissue.

Cortisone: a steroid hormone used to treat a variety of ailments by suppressing the immune system, thus reducing inflammation and attendant pain and swelling at the site of the injury.

Dermatology: the branch of medicine dealing with the skin and its diseases, a specialty with both medical and surgical aspects.

Erythema: redness of the skin, caused by increased blood flow through the capillaries in the lower layers of the skin.

Esthetician (or **aesthetician**): a licensed professional expert in maintaining and improving healthy skin, a practice generally limited to the epidermis (outer layer of skin).

Hyperpigmentation: the darkening of an area of skin or nails caused by increased melanin.

Laser: a device that emits light (electromagnetic radiation) through a process of optical amplification based on the stimulated emission of photons. Light propagates as waves and the "waves" emitted by a laser are said to be highly "coherent", that is, in step, and so more focused and powerful than ordinary light. Terms such as "CO_2 laser", "erbium laser" and so on refer to substances used to generate the laser beams and determine their various characteristics.

Melatonin: this so-called neurohormone is a naturally occurring compound whose many biological effects are produced through activation of melatonin receptors and through its role as a pervasive and powerful antioxidant. The best-known role of melatonin in humans is its regulation of the sleep-wake cycle.

Mohs surgery: microscopically controlled surgery used to treat common types of skin cancer. After each removal of tissue, while the patient waits, the pathologist examines the tissue specimen for cancer cells, and that examination informs the surgeon where to remove tissue next.

OBGYN: obstetrics and gynecology, the two surgical–medical specialties dealing with the female reproductive organs in their pregnant and non-pregnant state respectively, are often combined to form a single medical specialty and postgraduate training programme shortened to OB/GYN.

Photoaging: the characteristic skin changes induced by chronic exposure to ultraviolet (UVA and UVB) light.

Residency program: This is the graduate stage of medical training, wherein a physician practices medicine under the supervision of licensed physicians. Most residencies are performed in a hospital or clinic.

Resurfacing, ablative: This older technique uses mechanical abrasives to remove the upper layer of skin and so permit skin renewal.

Resurfacing, fractional laser: Employs heat induced by laser light to put tiny holes in the upper layers of the skin to stimulate the growth of new skin.

Rosacea: a chronic condition characterized by facial redness and sometimes pimples.

Scar, keloidal: A result of an overgrowth of granulation tissue at the site of a healed skin injury. Keloids are firm, rubbery lesions or shiny, fibrous nodules.

Scar, hypertrophic: A cutaneous condition characterized by deposits of excessive amounts of collagen, which gives rise to a raised scar, but not to the degree observed with keloids.

Silicone: silicones are polymer molecules that include the element silicon together with carbon, hydrogen, oxygen, and sometimes other elements. The medical grade gel form is used in breast and other implants and a variety of other medical uses.

Surgery, plastic: A surgical specialty dedicated to reconstruction of facial and body defects due to birth disorders, trauma, burns, and disease.

Surgery, cosmetic: A surgical specialty dedicated to enhancing a person's appearance toward some aesthetic ideal.

Surgery, vascular: A specialty of surgery in which diseases of the vascular system, or arteries and veins, are managed by medical therapy, minimally-invasive catheter procedures, and surgical reconstruction.

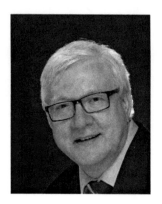

*D*r. Barry Lycka, based in Edmonton, Alberta, is widely acknowledged as one of North America's foremost authorities in cosmetic surgery and is the author of four best selling books: *Shaping A New Image, More Shaping, Restoring Youth,* and *SkinWorks.* He is Assistant Clinical Professor at the University of Alberta and has served as vice-president of the American Society of Cosmetic Dermatology and Aesthetic Surgery. He is the founder of Well and Wise Media Corporation and the Canadian Skin Cancer Foundation. He is host and founder of *YourCosmeticDoctor.tv* and host of *Inside Cosmetic Surgery Today* on WebTalkRadio.net. Dr. Lycka is a frequent guest speaker at international symposia and has presented recently at Sharm Derma in Cairo, Egypt and the Cosmetic Surgery Forum in Las Vegas, Nevada.

Dr. Lycka has won the Consumers Choice Award for Cosmetic Surgery for eleven consecutive years.

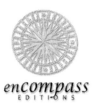

encompass
E D I T I O N S

ENCOMPASS EDITIONS, founded in 2009 and
based in Kingston, Ontario, Canada, is dedicated
to providing access to traditional publishing to a
wider spectrum of writers than is often the case—
writers in the United States, Canada, the United
Kingdom and the European Union. Although Encompass does not accept unsolicited manuscripts,
the company relies upon several agents who work
closely with writers of every level of experience. This
policy permits Encompass to focus on what it does
best: publish books good to read. You can visit the
Encompass website at www.EncompassEditions.
com or contact editor Robert Buckland at words@
encompasseditions.com

CPSIA information can be obtained at www.ICGtesting.com
Printed in the USA
BVOW081440110313

315231BV00001B/5/P